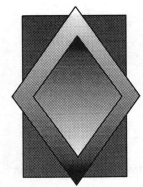

Instructor's Manual to Accompany

Community Health Nursing

Concepts And Practice

Fourth Edition

Barbara Walton Spradley, RN, MN
Judith A. Allender, RN, C, EdD

Prepared by
Judith A. Allender RN, C, EdD

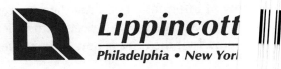 *Lippincott*

Philadelphia • New York

Sponsoring Editor: Susan M. Glover, RN, MSN
Editorial Assistant: Gene Bender
Ancillary Editor: Doris S. Wrey
Compositor: Richard G. Hartley
Printer/Binder: George H. Buchanan

Fourth Edition

0-397-55344-7

6   5   4   3   2   1

Any procedure or practice described in this book should be applied by the healthcare practitioner under appropriate supervision in accordance with professional standards of care used with regard to the unique circumstances that apply in each practice situation. Care has been taken to confirm the accuracy of information presented and to describe generally accepted practices. However, the authors, editors, and publisher cannot accept any responsibility for errors or omissions or for any consequences from application of the information in this book and make no warranty express or implied, with respect to the contents of the book.

Every effort has been made to ensure drug selections and dosages are in accordance with current recommendations and practice. Because of ongoing research, changes in government regulations and the constant flow of information on drug therapy, reactions and interactions, the reader is cautioned to check the package insert for each drug for indications, dosages, warnings and precautions, particularly if the drug is new or infrequently used.

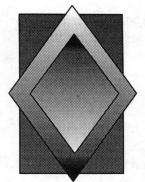

Preface

This Instructor's Manual is designed to assist nursing faculty using the text COMMUNITY HEALTH NURSING, Fourth Edition by Barbara W. Spradley, RN, MN and Judith A. Allender, RN, C, EdD. It provides suggestions for enhancing both classroom and clinical laboratory learning of community health concepts.

The chapters in this manual correlate with the chapters in the text. Each chapter includes learning objectives, key terms, a summary of the chapter concepts, teaching strategies to promote critical thinking in the classroom and clinical laboratory settings, and a variety of evaluation strategies.

Each chapter also contains the *learning objectives* and *key terms* found in the beginning of each textbook chapter. The learning objectives are stated in behavioral terms and reflect the most important concepts presented in the chapter. These objectives may be used by faculty in preparing course syllabi, lesson plans, or distributed as study guides for students. Key terms are identified to assist faculty in preparing classroom content or terminology worksheets for students.

The *chapter summary* highlights community health nursing content found in the 28 textbook chapters. The summary provides the faculty member with a quick review of major themes and concepts.

The *teaching strategies* section includes suggestions for both classroom and clinical laboratory teaching with a focus on enhancing critical thinking. The *classroom strategies* illustrate and amplify concepts presented in the text. A variety of suggestions are provided to give an educator latitude to choose those that seem most appropriate for his or her own group of students. The strategies include ideas for role play, simulation gaming, class discussion, group and individual activities, as well as suggestions for guest speakers and panel discussions by experts in the community. The *clinical laboratory strategies* provide ideas for experiential activities aimed at reinforcing classroom teaching and promoting critical thinking. Again, inclusion of a variety of experiences and settings gives faculty a wide choice when planning clinical activities.

The *evaluation strategies*, which stem from the learning objectives, consist of questions designed to promote critical thinking and evaluate students' understanding of the major concepts in each chapter. Evaluation strategies are presented through multiple choice, true/false, or essay questions and individual or group project ideas. They may be used to review content, as part of a formative evaluation, or as part of a formal examination for summative evaluation. Answers and rationales for the answer choices are provided in a separate answer section following Chapter 28.

I hope that faculty who use this manual along with COMMUNITY HEALTH NURSING, Fourth Edition, will find many ideas to help them develop creative teaching strategies and effective evaluation methods, thereby enhancing student learning.

I wish to acknowledge the people who have assisted in the preparation of this manual, especially my editor, Susan Glover, RN, MSN and the editing and design staff at Lippincott - Raven Publishers.

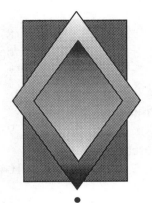

Table Of Contents

Unit Three: Promoting and Protecting the Health of Families

Unit Four: Promoting and Protecting the Health of Populations

Unit Five: Expanding the Community Health Nurse's Influence

Appendix A: Answers to Evaluation Questions

Conceptual Bases for Community Health Practice

Learning Objectives

- Discuss the concept of community.
- Identify three types of communities.
- Explain the wellness-illness continuum of health.
- Describe three distinguishing features about health.
- Differentiate between the three levels of prevention.
- Analyze six components of community health practice.
- Describe four characteristics of community health practice.

Key Terms

- Aggregate
- Common-interest Community
- Community
- Community Health
- Community of Solution
- Evaluation
- Geographic Community
- Health
- Health Continuum
- Health Promotion
- Illness
- Population
- Primary Prevention
- Public Health
- Rehabilitation
- Research
- Secondary Prevention
- Tertiary Prevention
- Wellness

Chapter Summary

The concepts of community and health are introduced in this chapter. A community is broadly defined as "a collection of people who share some important feature or features of their lives in common." Three types of communities are identified in relation to community health practice: geographic, common-interest, and a community of solution. The concern for groupings of people, as a unit of service, are a distinguishing feature of community health practice. The concepts of population and aggregates are also introduced as a foundation to community health practice and nursing.

The concept of health is described as relative rather than absolute, involving many levels of wellness or illness on a continuum. Health is always changing, moving back and forth along this continuum throughout the life of people and communities. Health is a state of being that involves the total person or total community. All aspects of life, including physical, psychological, sociocultural, and spiritual factors influence the health of an individual or a community. Health has both subjective and objective dimensions. The subjective dimension involves the level of well-being a person feels, and the objective dimension involves the ability to function, which is measurable.

Community health practice encompasses the concepts and principles of public health and is concerned with the promotion, protection, and preservation of the health of communities. Six basic elements of practice are incorporated in community health programs and services: 1) promotion of healthful living, 2) prevention of health problems, 3) treatment of disorders, 4) rehabilitation, 5) evaluation, and 6) research.

Community health practice emphasizes population-focused health care. The promotion of health and prevention of illness are first-order priorities. The treatment of disorders or unhealthy conditions and restoration of function, measurement and analysis of aggregates, and management of health services through the use of principles from management and organizational theory are also emphasized in community health practice.

Teaching Strategies

A. Classroom Strategies

1. Encourage students to identify their place on the wellness-illness continuum and discuss factors influencing their decision (Activities to Promote Critical Thinking in the text, #5, p. 20).

2. Using the categories of community discussed in this chapter, ask the students to categorize as many "communities" they can. Discuss why they fall into each category.

3. Identify an aggregate who shares an environmental concern such as a landfill, air pollution, sewage disposal site, or noise pollution. Plot the boundaries of this community-of-solution on a map. (Use a county or state map to show the overlapping of geographical boundaries.)

B. **Clinical Laboratory Strategies**

1. Use the Activities to Promote Critical Thinking statements # 1-4, p. 5 in the text to analyze the community served by the students in their community health clinical laboratory.
2. Have students choose one health practice of the college or university community to investigate, such as smoking habits, sleep habits, or dental practices. Help the students develop a tool to carry out a survey of the health practice. (Note: the appropriate human subjects' protections should be used.)
3. Have students analyze the data they have collected for frequency and percentage of students performing or not performing the identified health practice. Determine health promotion measures that would maintain or improve a healthy lifestyle.

Evaluation Strategies

A. **Multiple Choice Questions**

1. A community of solution is best described as a(n)
   a. community with well-defined geographical boundaries.
   b. a group of people who solve a problem that affects them.
   c. community with diverse members and interests within a defined area.
   d. location served by county and/or state health departments.

2. Rehabilitation
   a. focuses on health promotion and illness prevention.
   b. is an example of services provided during secondary prevention.
   c. takes corrective action to promote healthful living with a well population.
   d. focuses on reducing disability and restoring function.

3. Community health nursing students conducted a scoliosis screening program at a junior high school. This type of program is an example of
   a. primary prevention.
   b. secondary prevention.
   c. tertiary prevention.

4. A young couple's four-month-old infant died of Sudden Infant Death Syndrome (SIDS). The community health nurse encouraged the couple to join a SIDS support group. This activity is an example of
   a. primary prevention.
   b. secondary prevention.
   c. tertiary prevention.

5. A group of community residents sought a community health nurse's assistance/guidance in forming a community action group to investigate the impact that a proposed sanitary landfill would have on the health of their community. This is an example of
   a. primary prevention.
   b. secondary prevention.
   c. tertiary prevention.

B. True/False Questions

1. The terms, health and wellness, have subjective and objective dimensions.
   a. True
   b. False

2. Community health seeks to raise levels of wellness by achieving access to necessary prevention services for everyone.
   a. True
   b. False

3. Blood pressure screening offered by student nurses in a shopping mall is an example of primary prevention.
   a. True
   b. False

4. Student nurses, as a group, are considered a geographic community.
   a. True
   b. False

5. An aggregate focus is a distinguishing feature of community health practice.
   a. True
   b. False

C. Essay Questions

1. Design a health promotion program for yourself. Identify areas needing improvement in your health and make recommendations, outline goals, and include time lines for accomplishing this program.

2. Place the community you live in on the wellness-illness continuum. Why did you place it where you did? What areas need to be changed to move it to a higher level of wellness? What can YOU do about it as a community health nursing student?

D. Individual or Group Projects

1. Attend a city council or county board of supervisors meeting where legislators are discussing a community change which might affect the health of your community. Analyze how the changes may affect the community. If they allow discussion from citizens during the meeting, contribute your thoughts on the effects of the proposed change.

2. Identify a community problem that a group of student nurses in community health nursing clinical laboratory could solve. As a group, plan to solve the problem working with appropriate community members. Raise the needed funds, establish roles for each student, develop a time line, and complete the project. (As a record of the project, take a series of before and after photographs or photograph the event and give a set of photographs to the agency involved with the project.)

2

Structure and Function of Community Health Services

Learning Objectives

- Trace historic events and philosophy leading to today's health services delivery.
- Outline the current organizational structure of the public health care system.
- Describe the three core functions of public health.
- Differentiate between the functions of public versus private sector health care agencies.
- Explain the influence of selected legislative acts in the United States on shaping current health services policy and practice.

Key Terms

- Assessment
- Assurance
- Core public health functions
- Department of Health and Human Services
- Edwin Chadwick
- Hebrew hygienic code
- Medically indigent
- Official health agencies

- Pan American Health Organization
- Policy Development
- Proprietary health services
- Public Health Service
- Quarantine
- Sanitation
- Shattuck Report
- Voluntary health Agencies
- World Health Organization

Chapter Summary

Methods of delivering health care services to the public have evolved over time. Chapter 2 traces this evolution from ancient history to the present, then describes the current structure and functions of health service delivery systems in the United States. The chapter concludes with an overview of major legislative acts affecting the health of the nation and implications for community health nursing.

The first recorded public health efforts began as early as 3000 B.C. when inhabitants of ancient Egypt and the Middle East developed drainage systems and hygiene practices designed to preserve health. Concern for sanitation, hygiene, diet, and exercise lapsed during the Middle Ages, however, when people thought that disease was a punishment for sin and believed that pampering the body was evil. As a result, there were widespread outbreaks of disease. During the 1300s, bubonic plague reportedly killed 60 million people, half of the world's population (Hecker, 1839). In response to this, quarantine restrictions were enforced to prevent the spread of diseases. Health reforms were instituted in Europe at the end of the eighteenth century, fostered by a new interest in scientific investigation, human dignity, and human rights. During the nineteenth century, England led the way in public health. The first sanitary legislation was passed in 1837 in London. Edwin Chadwick's reform efforts led to the passage of the English Public Health Act and establishment of a General Board of Health for England in 1848.

In Colonial America through the late 1700s there was little effort made to protect the public's health. Public health in the United States began with efforts to control serious communicable diseases such as smallpox, cholera, and typhoid. Sanitary progress came about largely due to Lemuel Shattuck's 1850 report about health and sanitary problems in Massachusetts. Shattuck's report was the first to advocate the establishment of nurses' training, local boards of health, urban planning and preventative medicine among other public health related advances. However, American sanitary ordinances were patterned after well developed British laws.

This chapter describes the historic beginnings of community health programs, both public and private, and discusses the structure and aims of these systems. The three core functions of public health, assessment, policy development, and assurance are reviewed. Tax supported or governmentally administered health services are provided at four levels: local, state, national, and international. The four levels differ in structure and set of functions. The federal level of public health organization, the Public Health Service, is made up of six functional branches, such as the Centers for Disease Control and Prevention, the Food and Drug Administration, and the National Institutes of Health. At the international level, organizations such as the World Health Organization were developed to direct and coordinate the promotion of health worldwide.

In the private sector, organizations such as the American Cancer Society and the American Heart Association are voluntary non-profit organizations. Another group of private, not for-profit agencies affecting health and health care programs, research and professional education include agencies such as the W.K. Kellogg Foundation and the Pew Charitable Trust. For-profit proprietary groups also exist and are privately owned and operated. The private sector also includes professional services such as the practices of physicians, nurses, psychologists, social workers, and laboratory or technological services.

During the 20th century, in the United States, the financing and delivery of community health services widened with the passage of many important health related legislation. Over twenty of the most significant acts that took affect between 1921 and 1990 are discussed in this chapter. They have influenced health related concerns in areas such as maternal and child health, health insurance, prospective payment for health care, health planning facilities, Medicare and Medicaid.

A community health nurse's ties are very close to private and public health agencies, especially at the national, state, and local levels. Nurses have had to learn to adapt to a constantly changing system and be able to interpret current agency functions to clients and others. Collaboration with public and private agencies is important for nurses, in order to be able to promote quality and access to care in the broader community.

Teaching Strategies

A. Classroom Strategies

1. Lecturing on the important health service acts may not be effective. Have students research selected acts and report on them briefly, including an example of how the act has affected an individual or group.
2. Has a local agency lost funding or received additional funding? If so, discuss how this change will affect health locally or regionally.
3. Have a speaker from the local Social Security office speak to the class about services provided and the requirements that must be met for such services.

B. Clinical Laboratory Strategies

1. Have each student secure an organizational chart from a local health care agency. The students should identify the type of agency and compare and contrast the effectiveness of the structures.
2. Have each student visit a health service agency in the community and describe the function of that agency, the population served and its type (i.e., a private practice,

private proprietary agency, or voluntary agency). Compile a directory of these agencies for student reference.

3. If your students work in a health care agency during community health clinical laboratory, ask the supervising nurse to share the structure of the agency and how it "fits" into the local health care delivery system.

Evaluation Strategies

A. Multiple Choice Questions

1. Official health care agencies are
    - a. tax-supported.
    - b. voluntary.
    - c. proprietary.
    - d. privately-supported.

2. The level of health care agency where people actually receive their services is
    - a. international.
    - b. national.
    - c. state.
    - d. local.

3. The earliest recorded public health efforts can be traced back to
    - a. prehistoric centuries.
    - b. 3000 B.C.
    - c. 500 A.D.
    - d. 1800 A.D.

4. England led the way in public health and established a General Board of Health in the middle of the
    - a. 1200s.
    - b. 1400s.
    - c. 1600s.
    - d. 1800s.

5. An example of a voluntary agency is the
   a. American Red Cross.
   b. American Heart Association.
   c. National Institutes of Health.
   d. Public Health Service.

B. True/False Questions

1. In the 1800s, progress in health and sanitation came about largely due to the contributions of C. Everett Koop.
   a. True
   b. False

2. The three core functions of public health services are assessment, policy development, and assurance.
   a. True
   b. False

3. Voluntary health agencies are supported by private donations.
   a. True
   b. False

4. In the United States, there have been about five legislative acts in the 1900s shaping current health service policy and practice.
   a. True
   b. False

5. PL 98-21 changed the billing classification system to hospitals in 1983 in an attempt to control rising health care costs.
   a. True
   b. False

C. Essay Questions

1. Select a legislative act passed in the 1900s and discuss how the changes brought about by the act have affected you personally and professionally.

2. Describe what life might have been like 5000 years ago before the need for health care practices was recognized.

D. Individual or Group Projects

1. Have groups of students select a legislative act, research its development in depth, analyze it, and share opinions about it.

2. Have students write to their congressman or senator and share an opinion on a piece of legislation before the legislature at this time.

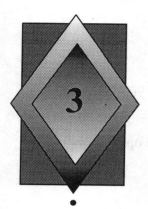

3

Health Care Economics

Learning Objectives

- Define the concept of health economics.
- Describe three sources of health care financing.
- Analyze the issues and trends influencing health care economics and community health services delivery.
- Explain the causes and effects of health care rationing.
- List the pros and cons of managed care competition as opposed to a single payer system.
- Explain the philosophical implications of heath care financing patterns on public health's mission and values.

Key Terms

- Competition
- Cost sharing
- Diagnosis-Related Groups
- Gross National Product
- Health economics
- Managed care
- Managed competition
- Medicaid
- Medicare
- National Health Insurance

- Preferred Provider Organization
- Prospective payment
- Rationing
- Regulation
- Retrospective payment
- Single payer system
- Third-party payments
- Universal coverage

Chapter Summary

This chapter presents a comprehensive discussion of the economic trends and issues that are now affecting health care delivery. The decisions and changes made today with our dwindling resources will affect our system long into the future. Production, distribution, and consumption of health care goods and services are studied in order to maximize the use of scarce resources and benefit the most people.

The influence of economic theories such as micro and macroeconomics as a foundation for health services delivery begins the chapter. The financing of health care through public and private sources fall into three categories, 1) third-party payers, 2) direct consumer payment, and 3) private support. Reimbursement for health care is made in two ways: after a service is rendered, retrospectively, or prospectively, through premiums paid in response to a fixed rate established by the provider. There is an incentive in prospective payment systems to contain costs but for some overzealous providers, clients are released from care in unstable conditions.

Regardless of the payment method, costs for health care have been growing at such a rate that services are being rationed in some states. Reasons for rising health care costs are many and too complex to solve simply. Inflation, complicated third-party reimbursement systems, the practice of defensive medicine and malpractice insurance, and a mood of unlimited spending are some of the major contributors.

Cost containment strategies have been tried since the 1970s, at first focusing on regulation and planning. In the 1980s the focus was on competition. Throughout the 1990s and into the 21st century, other methods such as cost sharing, self-insuring, and managed care will be the strategies implemented by health services agencies. Unfortunately, because of the rising cost of health care insurance, fewer and fewer employers are covering their employees, making health care inaccessible. Cutting costs at the expense of citizens is not the answer.

Health care reform has been talked about, argued about, and not universally agreed upon by those in decision making positions. However, managed care models have been growing and may be a compromise Americans can live with. Health maintenance and preferred provider organizations are two examples of alternative health care delivery systems under the managed care model. Other health care reform attempts under the managed care umbrella include managed competition and universal coverage within a single payer system. The universal coverage system discussed is similar to the Canadian system and is not without its problems. Consumers and professionals agree that health reform is needed in the U.S. but controversy surrounds what form it should take. Analyzing the systems in use in other countries may prove helpful.

Our country's health economics have seriously affected community health practice by advancing disincentives for efficient use of resources, incentives for illness care and conflict with public health values. A lack of spending limits encourages spending which drives up costs. Traditionally our system inadvertently tends to promote illness because providers have been rewarded for illness care and not preventative care.

Finally, our current health care model is present-oriented and focuses on individuals and illnesses. Public health is future-oriented, concerned with aggregates, and emphasizes prevention. This difference in focus makes it difficult for public health to remain competitive in a competitive health care system. In order for public health practice to be effective it needs to be excluded from health care competition, be free of unreasonable constraints, and receive dependable financial support in order to maintain organizational viability.

Teaching Strategies

A. Classroom Strategies

1. Arrange a debate on the health care reform issue. Divide the class into debate teams, and set up a debate format that fits in with the time allowed. Allow some students to be the "audience". Their responsibility will be to ask both sides pertinent questions at the end of the debate.

2. Invite the director of nursing from a home health agency to discuss how health care economics affects the functioning of a home health agency.

B. Clinical Laboratory Strategies

1. Invite the director of nursing from the agency where the students have their community health nursing laboratory to talk on health economics and how it affects public health practices locally.

2. Ask the students to assess their clients' health care insurance coverage. What type of system is it (public, private, HMO, PPO)? How does the family feel about it? Does it meet their needs? What would they change if they could?

Evaluation Strategies

A. Multiple Choice Questions

1. The following is true about Health Maintenance Organizations:
   a. they have a prospective payment system.
   b. they are a new model of managed care.
   c. billing paperwork remains expensive.
   d. about 5% of the U.S. population is enrolled

2. The following is true about Medicare:
   a. it covers about 25% of the U.S. population.
   b. both parts A and B have a fee involved.
   c. it covers most of the health care costs.
   d. it's a federal health insurance for elderly.

3. The following is true about Medicaid:
   a. it costs about $30 a month per person.
   b. the program is administered by each state
   c. it does not include preventative services.
   d. eligibility is determined by age and sex.

4. National Health Insurance
   a. has been adopted and it started in 1995.
   b. is not desired by the United States.
   c. has been debated for almost a century.
   d. is for those over 65 and disabled.

5. Health care economics as a concern for a community health nurse is
   a. something foreign and left to other members of the health care team.
   b. new and confusing and an issue for those in organizational management.
   c. important to the practice setting and for agency survival.
   d. mainly of utmost importance to the inservice educator in an agency.

B. True/False Questions

1. A HMO uses a prospective payment method.
   a. True
   b. False

2. Public health practice is highly competitive with private health care systems.
   a. True
   b. False

3. Medicare and Medicaid can be considered single payer systems.
   a. True
   b. False

4. Health care rationing has been talked about but is not being practiced in the United States.
   a. True
   b. False

5. Retrospective payment systems contribute to cost containment.
   a. True
   b. False

C. Essay Questions

1. You have the power to finance our health system. Give examples of changes you would make. How would these changes be financed?

2. Compare and contrast the services of a private physician and an HMO. Which do you prefer? Why?

D. Individual or Group Projects

1. Suggest that the students write to their congressman on a health care financing or health care reform issue.

2. Have groups of students work on Essay question number 1 as a group project.

4

Community Health Nursing: Past and Present

Learning Objectives

- Describe the four stages of community health nursing development.
- Analyze the impact of societal influences on community health nursing.
- Describe the primary characteristics of systems and adaptation theories as they relate to community health nursing practice.
- Explain the purpose and describe the variables that make up the conceptual framework for community health nursing presented in this chapter.
- Summarize the focus and nursing goals associated with the nursing models of Neuman, Orem, Pender, Roy, and Rogers.
- Explain six characteristics of community health nursing.

Key Terms

- Adaptation theory
- Collaboration
- Community health nursing
- Community health nursing dynamics
- Conceptual framework
- Coping mechanisms
- Health determinants
- Homeostasis
- Model
- Population-focused

- Practice interventions
- Practice priorities
- Public health nursing
- Scope of practice
- Self-care
- Stress
- Stressor
- System
- Systems theory
- Wellness

Chapter Summary

Community health nursing is a specialized nursing practice. The two characteristics of any specialized nursing practice are 1) specialized nursing knowledge and skills, and 2) a particular focus on the characteristics of the set of people receiving the service. Both are true for community health nursing. As health care continues to move out of the acute care setting many nurses from other specialties now practice in the community. It requires not only a shift from where the nurses practice, but also a shift in focus from individuals to aggregates.

The history of community health nursing developed in 4 general stages. Over the years community health nursing has evolved from early home care (before the mid 1880s), through district nursing (1860-1900), and public health nursing (1900-1970), to community health nursing (1970-present). Many contributions by nursing leaders are cited from the earliest days with Phoebe mentioned in the Bible as the first visiting nurse to the very significant contributions of Lillian Wald in the early 1900s. This was followed by formal recognition of public health nursing through the expansion of community health nursing settings and the subsequent growth of various nursing organizations that include and/or focus on public health nursing. It was during this time that the family emerged as the unit of service. By the 1970s the emergence of the term community health nursing heralded a new era. It began an era of other nurses beginning to practice in the growing numbers and kinds of settings in the community.

The growth of community health nursing was a result of six significant factors: advancements in technology, progress in causal thinking, changes in education, the changing role of women, the consumer movement, and economic factors. In this text the terms public health nursing and community health nursing are used interchangeably and refer to specialized population-focused nursing practice where public health and nursing principles are applied. Throughout the development of community health nursing it is evident how nurses in this specialty have provided leadership in planning and developing programs, in shaping policy, in administration, and in the application of research to promote the health of communities.

Community health nursing utilizes systems theory as a base. Systems theory states that, "every living system is a whole and its wholeness is made up of interdependent parts in interaction," (von Bertanlanffy, 1968). Systems theory, including Betty Neuman's Health Care Systems Model, is discussed in this chapter along with four other nursing models that are particularly relevant to community health nursing. Rogers' Model of the Science of Unitary Man, Pender's Health Promotion Model, Roy's Adaptation Model, and Orem's Self-care Model are included. Each model is described with examples of how each can be applied in the community.

The chapter concludes with a discussion of six major characteristics of community health nursing: 1) it is a field of nursing; 2) it combines public health with nursing; 3) it is population-focused; 4) it emphasizes wellness; 5) it involves interdisciplinary collaboration; and 6) it promotes individual, or aggregate, client responsibility and self-care.

Teaching Strategies

A. Classroom Strategies

1. Trace the history of community health nursing and discuss the confusion that has arisen about the definitions of community health nursing and public health nursing.

2. Ask the students to choose one of the five nursing models to describe their family as a system.

B. Clinical Laboratory Strategies

1. Use the Neuman health care systems model to guide the students in completing a community assessment of the community they serve in the community health clinical laboratory, are most personally familiar with, or the college or university community.

2. As a part of the students' community health clinical laboratory experience, discuss (during a clinical conference) how the students have seen the 6 characteristics of community health nursing demonstrated by the agency and nursing staff.

Evaluation Strategies

A. Multiple Choice Questions

1. From 1970 to the present, public health nursing has been termed community health nursing. Which of the following contributed MOST to this change?
   a. Decisions made by the American Nurses' Association
   b. The settings and nurses delivering health care in the community
   c. Decisions made by physicians in a variety of community settings
   d. The politics in the country and a desire to eliminate the word 'public'

2. The first person in recorded history to deliver nursing care in the home was mentioned in the Bible. Her name was
   a. Clarabelle.
   b. Sophie.
   c. Phoebe.
   d. Diana.

3. The characteristics of community health nursing include
   a. wellness.
   b. holism.
   c. dependency.
   d. individualism.

4. A nursing model that focuses on self-care is the model proposed by
   a. Rogers.
   b. Roy.
   c. Orem.
   d. Pender.

5. In Neuman's systems model the concept of homeostasis is discussed. This is best defined as
   a. a state of decline and deterioration.
   b. gender differences in clients.
   c. sexual preferences among humans.
   d. a state of equilibrium between parts.

B. True/False Questions

1. In Neuman's health care systems model *agitators* from the internal and external environment impact the health of clients.
   a. True
   b. False

2. In Orem's self-care model the goal is to promote people's collective independence and self-care ability.
   a. True
   b. False

3. Rogers developed her model around open systems, energy fields, patterns and organization, and four dimensionality.
   a. True
   b. False

4. Pender suggests that as people move toward healthier living there is a greater chance of healthy behaviors occurring.
   a. True
   b. False

5. In Roy's model, she suggests that people's adaptation levels are constant and stay the same throughout life.
   a. True
   b. False

C. Essay Questions

1. You are a nursing colleague of Lillian Wald. Imagine what nursing in New York City at the turn of the 20th century was like? Describe how it feels to be a nurse at that time.

2. Using one of the 5 nursing models discussed in this chapter as your conceptual framework, describe how you would provide care to an elderly couple with chronic illnesses, that is managing to live independently.

D. Individual or Group Projects

1. Have groups of five students design care for a hypothetical family. Each student should select a different nursing model. Compare and contrast the care plans and discuss the different foci of care.

2. Offer the opportunity for students to select a community health nurse from history and research his/her life and works. Students may select the nurse based on race, culture, location, or time in history. Allow classtime for sharing brief summaries of the nurses' works and times.

Roles and Settings for Community Health Nursing Practice

Learning Objectives

- Describe and differentiate between seven different roles enacted by community health nurses.
- Explain the importance of each role for influencing people's health.
- Identify and discuss factors that affect nurses' selection and practice of roles.
- Describe six settings in which community health nurses practice.
- Discuss the nature of community health nursing, the common threads basic to its practice, woven throughout all roles and settings.

Key Terms

- Advocate
- Case Management
- Clinician
- Collaborator
- Conceptual concepts
- Controller
- Educator

- Evaluator
- Human skills
- Leader
- Manager
- Planner
- Researcher
- Technical skills

Chapter Summary

Community health nurses have always practiced in a wide variety of settings and assumed various roles. In this chapter the seven major roles and six of the most common settings for CHN practice are examined. The seven major roles of the community health nurse are 1) clinician, 2) educator, 3) advocate, 4) manager, 5) collaborator, 6) leader, and 7) researcher.

The role of clinician or care provider is a familiar one for most people. In community health the clinician views clients in the context of larger systems. The family or group must be considered in totality. The community health nurse provides care along the entire range of the wellness-illness continuum; however, promotion of health and prevention of illness are emphasized. Skills in observation, listening, communication, counseling, and physical care are important for the community health nurse. Recent concerns for environmental, sociocultural, psychological, and economical factors in community health care have created a need for stronger skills in assessing the needs of populations at the community level.

One of the major functions of the community health nurse is that of health educator. As educators, nurses seek to facilitate client learning on a broad range of topics. They may act as consultants to individuals or groups, hold formal classes, or share information informally with clients. Self-care concepts, techniques for preventing illness, and health promotion strategies are emphasized throughout the health teaching process. (Chapter 14 discusses health teaching in greater depth.)

Two underlying goals in client advocacy are described. One goal of the community health nurse as advocate is to help clients find out what services are available, which ones they are entitled to, and how to obtain these services. A second goal is to influence change and make the system more relevant and responsive to clients' needs. Four characteristics required for successful advocacy are 1) assertiveness, 2) willingness to take risks, 3) good communication and negotiation skills, and 4) ability to identify resources and obtain results.

The manager's role is common to all nurses. Nurses serve as managers when they oversee client care, supervise ancillary staff, do case management, run clinics, or conduct community health needs assessment projects. The nurse engages in the four steps of the management process of planning, organizing, leading and controlling/evaluation. Each of these functions is described in the text. Specific decision-making behaviors are part of the manager's role as well as human, conceptual, and technical skills.

Collaboration with clients, other nurses, physicians, social workers, physical therapists, nutritionists, attorneys, secretaries, and other colleagues is part of the role of a community health nurse. Collaboration is defined as working jointly with others in a common endeavor to cooperate as partners. Skills required for successful collaboration are 1) communication skills, 2) assertiveness, and 3) consultant skills.

The role of leader is distinguished from the role of manager. As a leader, the community health nurse directs, influences, or persuades others to effect change that will positively affect people's health. Acting as a change agent and influencing health planning at the local, state, and national level are elements of the role of leader.

In the role of researcher, community health nurses engage in systematic investigation, collection, and analysis of data to enhance community health practice. (The research process is discussed in depth in Chapters 12 and 26.) Research in community health may range from simple inquiries to complex agency or organizational studies. Attributes of a nurse researcher include a questioning attitude, careful observation, open-mindedness, analytical skills, and tenacity.

Settings for community health nursing practice can be grouped into six categories: 1) homes, 2) ambulatory services settings, 3) schools, 4) occupational health settings, 5) residential institutions, and 6) the community at large. Each of these settings is described in this chapter.

The home has been the most frequently used site for community health nursing practice. In this setting the nurse has an opportunity to work with clients in the environment where they are most comfortable. This is changing however, with shifting health economics (discussed in Chapter 3) and the increased demand for highly technical care in the home has created new roles for nurses in the home setting (see Chapter 22).

Ambulatory care settings may include clinics, migrant camps, Native American reservations, correctional facilities, children's day care centers, churches, and rural, underserved communities. All of the roles of the community health nurse may be used in ambulatory care settings.

Schools provide another major setting for community health nursing practice. The role of the community health nurse in schools, from pre-schools to universities, is expanding to include health education, collaboration, and client advocation. (The school nurse's role is discussed in greater depth in Chapter 19.)

Occupational health settings are an expanding area for community health nursing practice. Businesses and industries are expected to provide a safe and healthy environment for their workers. The nurses in these settings act as employee advocates, collaborators, leaders, and managers. (Chapter 20 describes the role of the nurse in occupational settings.)

Community health nursing practice is not limited to a specific area. Residential institutions can be settings in which the community health nurse practices. Facilities such as half-way houses, long term care facilities, camping programs, sheltered workshops, and group homes can be challenging and unique settings for the community health nurse to practice. However it is important to remember that community health nursing is a specialty of nursing defined by the nature of its practice not by its location, (Anderson and Meyer, 1985; Williams, 1992).

Teaching Strategies

A. Classroom Strategies

1. Invite a panel of community health nurses who practice in a variety of settings and assume various roles to speak to the class. Ask the nurses to discuss each of the seven major roles according to the importance that is placed on it in their particular setting. Allow time for questions from the students after the presentation.

2. Find some copies of old nursing journals (1925-1940) and share the role expectations of nurses working in the community 50 or more years ago with today's roles. Let the students do this activity in class or prepare your lesson plan from the old journals and lead the discussion yourself.

B. Clinical Laboratory Strategies

1. At their assigned clinical practice site, have the students examine the major roles needed by nurses practicing at that or similar settings.

2. During a clinical conference, near the end of the clinical laboratory experience, ask the students to share examples of how they carried out the major roles of community health nurses, using examples from the work they did during the course.

Evaluation Strategies

A. Multiple Choice Questions

1. Sarah Jeffery, a community health nurse, collected data for several months on the birth weights of newborns to mothers who smoked throughout their pregnancy. This is an example of which of the following roles?
   a. Collaborator
   b. Manager
   c. Researcher
   d. Clinician

2. Ms. Jeffery spends time as a community health nurse working with secretaries, police officers, social workers, and other nurses. This is an example of her role as
   a. collaborator.
   b. advocate.
   c. manager.
   d. leader.

3. When Ms. Jeffery leads informed childbirth programs for expectant parents this is a demonstration of the role of
   a. researcher.
   b. educator.
   c. manager.
   d. collaborator.

4. At times Ms. Jeffery makes home visits and holds immunization clinics for infants and children. This is an example of the role of
   a. educator.
   b. advocate.
   c. leader.
   d. clinician.

5. When Ms. Jeffery organizes her day, plans client care, and leads staff conferences, she is fulfilling the role of
   a. manager.
   b. advocate.
   c. collaborator.
   d. researcher.

B. True/False Questions

1. One of the goals of the advocacy role is to help clients gain greater independence.
   a. True
   b. False

2. The practice setting for the community health nurse is limited to homes, ambulatory care settings, schools, and occupational health settings.
   a. True
   b. False

3. Research is an investigative process, and from that perspective all community health nurses are researchers.
   a. True
   b. False

4. The role of leader is not distinguishable from the role of manager.
   a. True
   b. False

5. The community health nurse as a collaborator assumes the role of a partner to work jointly with others in a common endeavor.
   a. True
   b. False

C. Essay Questions

1. Select one of the seven major roles of the community health nurse and develop it fully, using client foci and services offered, similar to the clinical laboratory setting in which you have been working.

2. Select one of the six categories in which community health nurses practice and develop the nurse's role of EDUCATOR in this setting.

D. Individual or Group Projects

1. Have the students select a practice setting of their choice (be sure all settings are selected at least once) and observe a nurse in this setting. The student should be prepared to discuss the nurse's role during a class later in the course.

2. Have the students identify the major employers in the community where the nursing program is located. Select the top 10 employers that do not have an occupational health nurse. Have small (2-3) groups of students meet with the safety director, public relations representative, or manager. Ask the company representative questions what they think a nurse could do for their company if they employed one. If the response is limited, the students should inform the representative what a nurse could do for the company. Use the seven major roles to build examples. Report the responses to the class.

Environmental Health and Safety

Learning Objectives

- Discuss the significance of systems theory and an ecological perspective on understanding human-environment relationships.
- Explain the concepts of prevention and long-range environmental impact and their importance for environmental health.
- Identify at least six areas of environmental health concern to community health nursing and describe the hazards associated with each area.
- Relate the effect of the above hazards on people's health.
- Discuss appropriate interventions for addressing the above environmental health problems including community health nursing's role.
- Identify at least six national health objectives for the year 2000 targeted at environmental health.
- Describe strategies for nursing collaboration and participation in efforts to promote and protect environmental health.

Key Terms

- Contaminant
- Ecological perspective
- Ecosystem
- Environment
- Environmental health

- Environmental impact
- Hazard
- Pollution
- Toxic Agents
- Vectors

Chapter Summary

Because environmental conditions strongly influence people's health status, the study of environmental health has tremendous meaning for the community health nurse. People's health and well-being are influenced by chemical, physical, and psychological forces that are present in their workplaces, home, and the larger community. The study of environmental health has become more complex as people's ability to influence their environment has increased. Determining environmental health means more that looking for illness or disease-causing agents. Health practitioners need to determine all the links between people and the environment in order to improve the health and well-being of both. In addition, it is essential to determine how current practices, policies, and substances are harming present and future generations.

Although many of the earliest environmental hazards have been eliminated through improved technology, many new and more complex hazards have been created. The historical development of health and safety laws established to control the quality of air, water, food and drugs, and improve safety in the workplace are reviewed. Because community health nurses may be called on to assess environmental health hazards, they need a general knowledge of how people's health is affected by toxic agents carried through air, water, food, vectors (rodents and insects), wastes, and the risks to health when safety is compromised in the home, worksite, and community. These six areas are discussed thoroughly in this chapter and include the government's and nurses' role for each area.

Air quality has affected human health for centuries and is now recognized as one of the most hazardous sources of chemical contamination. Due to industrial and auto emissions, thermal atmospheric inversions, and agricultural pesticides, serious life and health threatening air pollution has increased in recent years.

Water is an essential element to human survival and a prime environmental health issue. Having an adequate source of pure drinkable water has been of concern to humans throughout history. Major outbreaks of diseases have been linked to a contaminated water supply.

The presence of infectious agents in food is often underestimated. Food-borne infections and poisonings may cause more short-term illness than the common cold, and many instances of food-borne diseases have been made public in recent years. Three types of hazardous foods exist as possible health problems; 1) inherently harmful foods, such as certain mushrooms; 2) food contamination by chemicals or harmful bacteria such as salmonella; and 3) chemical additives such as red dye #2, preservatives, and artificial flavorings.

Insects and rodents living in a human environment are a nuisance and may cause economic loss and create health hazards, the most serious of which is through their role as vectors. The most common vectors are mosquitos, flies, ticks, roaches, fleas, rats, mice, and ground squirrels. Table 6-2 (text, p. 133) summarizes some of the disease spread by vectors.

Waste is another area of concern in environmental health. Personal and industrial waste generates almost 3500 pounds of waste per year per person in the United States (Moeller, 1992). It is imperative that health officials, including community health nurses, be aware of the possible health hazards these wastes present to individuals and to the community. Human waste provides a perfect environment in which bacteria and disease-causing parasites can live. Dumps provide a breeding ground for vectors and take up valuable land resources. Burning produces odors and air pollution. Landfills can contaminate ground water. More emphasis needs to be placed on recycling to reduce the amount of waste generated. Health threats are also created by the disposal of hazardous and toxic industrial waste products.

Safety in the home, worksite, and community environment is imperative for the protection of all ages. Exposure to toxic chemicals, radiation, injury from the risks of vehicular accidents, falls, drownings, poisonings, residential fires, violence, and psychological hazards are environmental safety issues from which people need protection through regulation and education.

The government's role in environmental health takes the form of establishing standards, enacting laws, regulating, inspecting and licensing. The community health nurse's role includes observing, detecting, reporting, teaching, informing the public, and conducting and applying research. Together the government, through state and local agencies, and the community health nurse collaborate to enhance and protect the environment for its human inhabitants.

Teaching Strategies

A. Classroom Strategies

1. Invite an environmental engineer or a representative of the Environmental Protection Agency (EPA) or the Occupational Safety and Health Administration (OSHA) or other appropriate speakers from the local health department to speak to the class about environmental hazards in the community.
2. Assign the students to develop a home environmental hazards checklist.

B. Clinical Laboratory Strategies

1. Have the students conduct a windshield survey of a selected geographic area to identify environmental hazards. Assign the students to diverse geographical areas to make comparisons of the kinds of hazards present (i.e., industrial, residential, commercial, rural, or high-density urban).

2. During a home visit to an assigned client ask the students to assess the home environment for obvious health hazards, using the checklist that was developed as a class assignment.

Evaluation Strategies

A. **Multiple Choice Questions**

1. An ecological perspective of environmental health is
    a. the study of governmental and private sector regulation of the environment.
    b. a technological view of strategies for preventing illness and injury.
    c. the role of the community health nurse in preventing disease and illness.
    d. the recognition that we affect the environment and the environment affects us.

2. A vector is defined as
    a. nonhuman carriers of disease organisms that can transmit disease directly to humans.
    b. a chemical, either natural or synthetic, which is capable of acting as a carcinogen.
    c. an infectious agent carried to humans through food sources.
    d. toxic substances introduced by humans into the underground water supply.

3. The issue of water pollution is
    a. a new one due to the proliferation of industries in the United States.
    b. a major problem in other countries, but not the United States.
    c. nonexistent in ground water sources, the use of which should be increased.
    d. significant because it causes millions of episodes of disease in the country each year.

4. The EPA was established in 1971, mainly to
    a. give authority over environmental issues.
    b. identify and address world health issues.
    c. protect occupational safety and health.
    d. monitor food and drug production and availability.

5. The discarding of disposable diapers is a problem. One of the problems is that
   a. they make up 10% of municipal wastes.
   b. they take centuries to deteriorate in a landfill.
   c. 3 billion disposable diapers are discarded each year.
   d. a few people discard the diaper with the feces in the diaper.

B. True/False Questions

1. Radon gas exposure in homes has become a topic of concern in recent years.
   a. True
   b. False

2. Surface water has fewer contaminants in it than underground water sources.
   a. True
   b. False

3. Food is safe from contamination and is not a hazard to people's health.
   a. True
   b. False

4. Insects and rodents are of concern to environmental health mainly because they are vectors.
   a. True
   b. False

5. Solid wastes from individuals and industry amount to over 1 and 1/2 tons per person in the United States per year.
   a. True
   b. False

C. Essay Questions

1. Go through your home mentally and listing each room and your yard, identify all the potential environmental health hazards. Identify how you would make the needed changes.

2. Select an article researching an environmental health issue in a copy of the *American Journal of Public Health*. Copy the abstract and distribute it in class. Ask the students to write a reaction to the problem and the study and determine how the study could be replicated in your community.

D. Individual or Group Projects

1. Divide the class into six groups. Each group selects one of the six categories of environmental concern and researches it locally. Explore your city or county for strengths and weaknesses in each area. Report findings to the class.

2. Ask students to bring newspaper articles to class that report on local, regional or state environmental health issues and share them throughout the duration of the course. Allow a few minutes to discuss each article. This could be voluntary or tied in with a class participation grade.

7

Influence of Culture on Community Health

Learning Objectives

- Define and explain the concept of culture.
- Identify five characteristics shared by all cultures.
- Discuss the meaning of cultural diversity and its significance for community health.
- Describe the meaning and effects of ethnocentrism on community health nursing practice.
- Contrast the health-related values, beliefs, and practices of culturally diverse populations with those of a dominant US culture.
- Conduct a cultural assessment.
- Apply transcultural nursing principles in community health nursing practice.

Key Terms

- Cultural assessment
- Cultural diversity
- Cultural relativism
- Cultural self-awareness
- Cultural sensitivity
- Culture
- Culture shock
- Dominant values
- Enculturation
- Ethnic group
- Ethnicity
- Ethnocentrism
- Microculture
- Minority group
- Race
- Tacit
- Transcultural nursing
- Value

Chapter Summary

Culture is described in this chapter as ideas, values and behaviors that are shared by members of a society and that provide a design or "map" for living. Culture influences people's beliefs, thoughts, and actions. Community health nurses must understand and appreciate cultural diversity because culture affects all aspects of daily living. The behaviors that are directly related to health include child-rearing methods, eating habits, reactions to pain and illness, and ways of coping with stress.

In the United States there are more than 100 different ethnic groups, 50 of which are large groups. The largest groups are African-Americans, Hispanic-Americans, and Asian/Pacific Rim-Americans. Presently these groups make up 12, 9 and 3% of our population. It has been estimated that by the year 2050, Hispanic-Americans will represent 21% of the population, while African-Americans and Asian/Pacific Rim-Americans will be 15 and 10% of the population (Current Population Reports, 1992). Within the United States there are microcultures and subcultures, which are relatively large aggregates who share ethnicity, occupation, religion, geographic area, age, or sexual preference.

Nurses must recognize cultural differences as a first step toward cultural understanding. They are challenged to learn communication techniques that will bridge barriers created by cultural differences. Ethnocentrism, or the belief that one's own culture is best, can impede effective communication. To overcome ethnocentrism, nurses must learn to set aside biases and preconceptions and be able to see the value of other people's ways of life. Nurses must understand and explore patients' traditional health practices and be able to look objectively at their safety and effectiveness.

Culture is 1) learned; 2) integrated; 3) shared; 4) tacit; and 5) dynamic. These five characteristics are shared by all cultures and are especially pertinent to nursing's effort to improve community health. The process of learning about one's culture, called enculturation, enables a person to behave in ways that the person's society sees as fitting and appropriate. Because one of the characteristics of culture is that it is learned, people can relearn some aspects of culture and adopt new behaviors or values. Culture is an integrated whole: a complex assortment of thoughts, actions, traits, and customs. Culture is the product of aggregate behavior, not individual habit. Shared cultural values provide stability, security, and standards for behavior. Because values are more deeply rooted than individual behaviors, they change very slowly. Culture is tacit in that it provides a guide for human interaction that is mostly unexpressed at the unconscious levels and understood through unspoken cues. Culture is dynamic and undergoes change, often adding and deleting components. Innovative members within a cultural group can effect change and be willing to adopt new ways.

Selected clusters of cultural communities served by community health nurses are reviewed briefly in this chapter. Specific population characteristics are shared for Native Americans, African-Americans, Asian/Pacific Rim-Americans, and Hispanic-Americans as well as disadvantaged populations such as those with low income, the homeless, and physically or mentally challenged populations.

A community health nurse must follow five principles for an effective transcultural practice. 1)develop cultural self-awareness; 2) cultivate cultural sensitivity, 3) assess client group's culture; 4) show respect and patience while learning about other cultures, and; 5) examine culturally derived health practices.

Teaching Strategies

A. Classroom Strategies

1. Ask a representative from one of the cultural groups in the local community (or from the community health nursing class) speak to the class about various aspects of his or her culture. The Cultural Assessment Guide in Table 7-3, p. 164 could be used by the speaker (if provided).
2. Invite a panel made up of representatives of the cultural communities to class to speak. This group may also be helped by the Cultural Assessment Guide either in it's original form or a modified one.

B. Clinical Laboratory Strategies

1. Have students present a cultural assessment of their own family. To highlight their presentation suggest they bring photographs of their family members, such as parents, siblings, significant others, and their own children.
2. Have students complete a cultural assessment on one of their assigned families that represent a specific cultural community (a minority ethnic group, a family living in poverty, the disabled). Share with peers in a community health clinical laboratory conference, perhaps as part of a case study.

Evaluation Strategies

A. Multiple Choice Questions

1. In 1980 the Harvard Encyclopedia listed over 100 different ethnic groups living in America, 50 of which are of a significant size. What is the largest minority group in America today?
   a. Asian-Americans
   b. African-Americans
   c. Hispanic-Americans
   d. Native Americans

2. Which of the following groups is growing at a rapid rate and will be the largest non-white group in the United States by 2050?
   a. Asian-Americans
   b. African-Americans
   c. Hispanic-Americans
   d. Native Americans

3. An attribute of low income populations according to Strauss (1967) is that they live
   a. mostly for today, in the present.
   b. for the future, sacrificing today.
   c. in the past when times were better.
   d. as all others do, with a time frame balance.

4. Native American cultural similarities include
   a. a concern for the distant future.
   b. encouraging competition between people.
   c. using western medicine before traditional.
   d. respect increasing age and elders.

5. In the Interaction Model of viewing people with disabilities, a person with a disability is seen as
   a. deficient.
   b. different.
   c. abnormal.
   d. negative.

B. True/False Questions

1. Ethnocentrism is a way of viewing other cultures and valuing them.
   a. True
   b. False

2. Cultures are always changing, indicating they are dynamic.
   a. True
   b. False

3. A subculture is a small cultural group within large national societies.
   a. True
   b. False

4. A major health problem of Asian/Pacific Rim-Americans is diabetes mellitus.
   a. True
   b. False

5. A comfortable talking distance for Americans is 30 inches.
   a. True
   b. False

C. Essay Questions

1. Select one of the following cultural values: food, religion, parenting, or health practices. Compare and contrast your behavior/beliefs in the selected area with someone from a cultural group different than yours.

2. Select one category of the Cultural Assessment Guide (Table 7-3, p.164) and develop a response using the Sample Data ideas. Describe this data in relation to your family of origin and how you (as an adult) view the same category.

D. Individual or Group Projects

1. Plan a poster session in which each of the students will design a poster depicting aspects of one culture in the local community (Assign groups of students to do this if there are not enough cultures and subcultures to assign one to each student).

2. Plan a film festival. Have the students locate several good films depicting different cultures. Have a tasting party of ethnic food eaten by these groups.

Values and Ethical Decision Making in Community Health

8

Learning Objectives

- Describe the nature of values and value systems and their influence on community health.
- Identify personal and professional values that they bring to decision making with and for community clients.
- Articulate the impact of key values on professional decision making.
- Discuss the application of ethical principles to community health nursing decision making.
- Use a decision making process with and for community clients that incorporates values and ethical principles.
- Participate in discussions about ethical aspects of community health nursing practice as a member of an agency ethics committee.

Key Terms

- Autonomy
- Beneficence
- Egalitarian justice
- Equity
- Ethics
- Ethical decision making
- Ethical dilemma
- Fidelity

- Instrumental values
- Justice
- Moral
- Moral evaluations
- Nonmaleficence
- Respect
- Restorative justice
- Self-determination

- Terminal values
- Values
- Values clarification

- Values systems
- Veracity
- Well-being

Chapter Summary

Community health nurses' practice and decision making are strongly influenced by their values. This chapter explores the nature of values and value systems, the role that values play in decision making and health care choices, and the implications for nursing practice.

Values serve as the criteria or standards by which judgements and decisions are made. The nature of values can be described according to five qualities: endurance, hierarchical system, prescriptive-proscriptive beliefs, reference, and preference. Values endure and provide continuity to personal and social existence. Value systems are generally considered organizations of beliefs that are of relative importance in guiding an individual's behavior. Values function as standards of behavior, while value systems function as plans for conflict resolution and decision making. Internalized values function as standards that guide personal conduct and moral judgements, and give expression to human needs.

Techniques for clarifying values can help people to find out how their own value system influences their behavior and decision making. Values clarification is a process that helps one identify the significant values that guide one's actions. The process of valuing involves steps such as choosing a value freely from alternatives, affirming the value, incorporating the value into a behavioral standard, and then consciously using the value in decision making.

Ethical decision making means making a choice that is consistent with a moral code or that can be justified from an ethical perspective. Any decision in nursing practice that involves a conflict over values may involve a moral conflict. Several frameworks for ethical decision making are presented in the text.

Three basic human values are considered key to guiding decision making in the provider-client relationship. They are self-determination, well-being, and equity. Self determination is a person's exercise of the capacity to shape and pursue personal plans for life. Well-being is a state of positive health or people's perception concerning positive health. Equity means being treated equally or fairly and having access to an adequate level of medical care. Seven fundamental ethical principles should guide community health nurses when making decisions: respect, autonomy, beneficence, nonmaleficence, justice, veracity, and fidelity (Aroskar, 1995; Jenkins, 1989). The ANA Code for Nurses with Interpretive Statements (1985) can be a helpful guide for community health nurses.

Teaching Strategies

A. Classroom Strategies

1. Assign the students to complete the Activities to Promote Critical Thinking in the text prior to the lecture/discussion of this chapter. Ask for volunteers to share their responses. (Note: Be prepared to give examples of typical responses if the students choose to share in a limited fashion.)

2. Provide the students with a brief case study that involves making an ethical decision. Find examples from the national or local media. Some situations have been in the media for months and serve as extreme examples.

B. Clinical Laboratory Strategies

1. Have the students identify actual or potential situations that could require the need for ethical decision making. Ask students to briefly describe one situation in their clinical journal (log or diary) or share one verbally in clinical conference.

2. Ask students to discuss with a trusted peer or community health nurse how the key values of self-determination, well-being, and equity guide her or his decision making in practitioner-client relationships.

Evaluation Strategies

A. Multiple Choice Questions

1. Prescriptive-proscriptive beliefs
   a. are nonmoral evaluations.
   b. determine if an action is desirable.
   c. refer to modes of conduct.
   d. are organized into a hierarchical system.

2. Which of the five qualities describing the nature of values explains that values guarantee stability in personal and social existence?
   a. endurance
   b. relativity
   c. reference
   d. preference

3. One of the basic human values that guides decision making is equity. This value is defined as
    a. the capacity to form, revise, and pursue personal life plans.
    b. interventions to promote clients' health and sense of well-being.
    c. the belief that like cases should be treated alike, and/or treated fairly.
    d. the preference for joint decision making over individual decision making.

4. The outcome of the basic human value of self-determination that can be expected is
    a. individual autonomy.
    b. a lowered self-concept.
    c. detrimental health behaviors.
    d. a lack of quality care.

5. The ANA Code for Nurses gives
    a. mandates to follow if you are a professional.
    b. rules that need to be followed to maintain licensure.
    c. guidelines to follow as practice is conducted ethically.
    d. moral judgments and outcomes of negative actions.

B. True/False Questions

1. Values clarification is a process of discovery of the values and underlying motivations that guide one's actions.
    a. True
    b. False

2. The process of valuing utilizes strategies to make judgmental decisions.
    a. True
    b. False

3. Values clarification strategies can be used to analyze how values ultimately influence people's behavior.
    a. True
    b. False

4. Ethics involves making evaluative judgements.
    a. True
    b. False

5. When judgements involve moral values, conflicts never occur.
    a. True
    b. False

C. Essay Questions

1. Provide the students with a short case study which involves an ethical dilemma and ask them to react to it in writing. Ask that the responses be anonymous. Read the responses and ask for class reactions to the various views shared. (This is a good exercise to stimulate thought, discussion and participation, not to be graded.)

2. Ask students to share an ethical dilemma they were part of or witnessed in their personal or professional life. How did they respond to it? How would they respond to it if it were to occur today? Is their response different now? Why?

D. Individual or Group Projects

1. Have the students participate in a debate. Follow a pre-determined debate format that you select. Allow the students to choose topics appropriate to community health nursing that are currently controversial within the profession. Have peers grade each group. Rationales for the grade should be given based on criteria you established.

2. Select item number 3 from the Activities to Promote Critical Thinking for this chapter. Have students rank the 12 items individually, allowing 5-7 minutes for the exercise. Then suggest that students work in small groups (select the groups by birthday months or counting off by 5s, or use some system so clusters of friends may be in different groups) for 15 minutes to come up with a common ranking reached by consensus. Discuss the difficulty of the individual task versus the group task. What items created the greatest concession for students? Why? Why did they concede so much?

The Community as Client: Assessment and Planning

9

Learning Objectives

- Explain why nurses must move beyond an individualistic focus to practice population-based community health nursing.
- Describe the meaning of community as client.
- Articulate specific considerations of each of the three dimensions of the community as client.
- Express the meaning and significance of community dynamics.
- Explain four types of community needs assessment.
- Discuss community needs assessment methods.
- Describe characteristics of a healthy community.
- Identify the steps in planning for the health of a community.

Key Terms

- Client myth
- Community
- Community as client
- Community needs assessment
- Community subsystem assessment
- Comprehensive assessment
- Descriptive epidemiological study
- Familiarization assessment
- Individualism
- Location myth
- Location variables
- Population variables
- Problem-oriented assessment
- Skills myth
- Social class
- Social system variables
- Survey

Chapter Summary

Three pervasive myths have hindered nurses from focusing on aggregate care: the location myth, the skills myth, and the client myth. The location myth defines community health nursing in terms of where it is practiced such as outside the hospital setting. The skills myth states that community health nurses employ only the skills of basic clinical nursing in work with community clients. The client myth says that the primary clients are individuals and families. All three myths are perpetuated by the high value that people in the United States place on individualism.

In this text, community health nursing's primary mission of working with communities at six levels is described as practice with and for the community. It involves individuals, family, groups, subpopulations, populations and communities. Nursing practice employs nursing expertise together with skills and concepts from public health.

In assessing the health of a community, nurses must have a three-dimensional view of the community as client. The location dimension involves variables such as boundaries, location of health services, geographic features, climate, flora and fauna, and human-made environment. The population dimension focuses on aspects such as size, density, composition, growth rates, cultural characteristics, educational level and social class, and mobility. The social system dimension examines roles, organizations, and interacting subsystems within a community. The health care system as a part of a community is of particular importance to the community health nurse.

Conceptual frameworks and models can enhance the planning for community health programs. In addition, aggregate level teamwork with other professionals as well as with clients are community health nursing practice considerations.

Community dynamics, described as the driving forces that govern a community's functioning, are influenced by two factors in particular; citizen participation and power and decision making structure. When community members participate actively in community decision making, the community is capable of self care. However, the power and decision making structure of a community is of central concern when anyone desires to bring about change.

A community's needs can be assessed in several ways. A comprehensive assessment seeks to discover all relevant community health information. A familiarization assessment relies primarily on existing data, supplemented with some information gained first-hand. To gain a working knowledge of the community, a problem-oriented assessment begins with a single problem and assesses the community in terms of that problem. A community subsystem assessment focuses on a single dimension of community life. Surveys and descriptive epidemiologic studies are two methods of conducting community assessments.

To be healthy, a community must be able to collaborate effectively in identifying needs and problems, to achieve a working consensus on goals and priorities in problem-solving, with ways and means to implement a plan to achieve the goals, and to collaborate effectively on the required actions.

Community assessment is the foundation on which a community health planning process is formulated. A four-stage process is proposed for community health planning and includes assessment, analysis and design, implementation, and evaluation stages. The nursing process detailed in Chapter 11 becomes an important tool to facilitate nursing practice with the community as client.

Teaching Strategies

A. Classroom Strategies

1. Obtain copies of various individual and family assessment tools used by nurses practicing in a variety of settings. Compare the tools and discuss the merits of each.

2. Designate a locale familiar to all students (such as their own home town or the college campus) and have students use the Community Profile Inventory (p. 193) to assess and identify sources of information. Have students use the questions from the Community Profile to develop an assessment of their community from the dimensions of location, population, and social system.

B. Clinical Laboratory Strategies

1. Using the information gathered in classroom strategies #1, design a tool to use in the clinical laboratory (do this in conjunction with clinical laboratory site staff). Pilot the tool, make necessary changes and suggest the staff use the tool if they find it helpful.

2. Identify the census tracts of the city in which the students have their clinical laboratory experience. Have groups of students conduct a comprehensive community assessment of each census tract using the Community Profile Inventory on p.193. Share the findings during a clinical conference.

Evaluation Strategies

A. Multiple Choice Questions

1. Population-focused practice is best described by which of the following nursing activities?
   a. Assisting a workman injured in an industrial accident.
   b. Checking a school-child's hair for lice
   c. Speaking to county commissioners about the need for additional senior services
   d. Counseling a young man about safe sex and HIV/AIDS

   The following situation applies to questions 2 through 4:

   The nursing student in a community heath nursing course identified toxic waste disposal to be a major problem in their community.

2. The most cost-effective type of community assessment to determine the extent of the problem and the resources available to handle it would be a
   a. familiarization assessment.
   b. problem-oriented assessment.
   c. community subsystem assessment.
   d. comprehensive community assessment.

3. The students conducted a survey to determine community awareness of the problem of toxic waste disposal. The final and most important step in conducting a survey is to
   a. develop the survey questionnaire or interview guide.
   b. process data and determine relationships.
   c. report the implications and recommendations of the survey results.
   d. collect data using a valid and reliable tool.

4. The data obtained from the community assessment and survey was used as the basis for developing a health program. A good way to implement the program would be to
   a. plan a clean-up committee made up of students.
   b. petition the state government about the danger of genetic problems.
   c. ask the city council to hold a town meeting to discuss the problem.
   d. write to a local news station or "60 Minutes" for public disclosure.

5. You are part of a health planning team to determine the needs of the pregnant teenagers in your community. Which of the following population variables would you want to assess?
   a. Location of health services
   b. Functions of community organizations
   c. Health needs and practices of subcultural groups
   d. Level of agreement on community goals

B. True/False Questions

1. A "Windshield Survey" is an example of a comprehensive community assessment.
   a. True
   b. False

2. The "location myth" defines a nurse's practice on the location of its delivery.
   a. True
   b. False

3. There are two levels of clients in a community health nurse's scope of practice.
   a. True
   b. False

4. The three dimensions of a community are location, population, and a social system.
   a. True
   b. False

5. In a problem-oriented assessment, a community is assessed in terms of that problem.
   a. True
   b. False

C. Essay Questions

1. Select one dimension of a community you are familiar with and, using the community assessment questions from Tables 9.2, 9.3, or 9.4, answer the questions in relation to the community selected.

2. Select a problem (other than child abuse) in the community. Identify the levels of prevention needed to reduce the incidence of this problem. Refer to the levels of prevention display on p. 207 for format.

D. Individual or Group Projects

1. Using classroom strategy #1 and clinical laboratory strategy #1, modify them to be an individual or group project in class or clinical laboratory.

2. Outline a strategy to assess a community using one of the needs assessment methods discussed in this chapter. Share your rationale for selecting the method chosen before outlining the steps you'll take.

10

Working with Populations and Groups

Learning Objectives

- Differentiate between five different kinds of groups with whom community health nurses work.
- Identify essential group needs.
- Describe the elements to be considered in starting a group.
- Explain the significance of group cohesiveness.
- Identify the phases of group development.
- Describe and practice group leader and member roles and functions.
- Assist a group through termination.
- Design both process and outcome evaluation of group goals.
- Differentiate between groups and populations.
- Articulate strategies for working with populations.
- Compare similarities in working with groups and populations.

Key Terms

- Counterdependence phase
- Dependence phase
- Group
- Group cohesiveness
- Interdependence phase
- Learning group
- Maintenance roles
- Outcome evaluation
- Population
- Process evaluation
- Psychotherapy group
- Socialization group
- Support group
- Task-oriented group
- Task roles

Chapter Summary

The community health nurse works with populations and groups of all sizes to promote the health of the community. The focus of this chapter is two-fold; to adopt an aggregate orientation for practice and to develop skills in working with aggregates. A group is defined as "a collection of persons who engage in repeated, face-to-face communication, identify with each other, experience interdependence, and share a common purpose or purposes".

In order to work effectively with a group, the community health nurse needs to know what kind of group it is, what its needs are, and what its major functions should be. The five types of groups most frequently encountered in community health nursing practice are listed below.

1. Learning groups, whose primary goal is for members to gain understanding in order to effect behavior change in some specified area of need.

2. Support groups, which aim to promote healthy behaviors and prevent maladaptive coping patterns among its members.

3. Socialization groups, which help members to learn new social roles in order to achieve a positive level of health.

4. Psychotherapy groups, which are formed to promote the health of people with an emotional disturbance.

5. Task-oriented groups, whose primary goal is to accomplish tasks towards meeting specified goals.

A small-group has four essential sets of needs that must be satisfied and maintained to function optimally. These include shared goals, consistent norms that govern the group's actions, motivated participants, and stable channels of communication. The primary functions of a group can be divided into task-related functions and group maintenance functions. A well-functioning group will succeed in achieving a balance between the task and maintenance concerns.

Criteria for membership in a group and the optimal number of members are primary considerations when establishing a group. The needs of the client and the task of the group should be considered when determining group size. Establishing group goals, making physical arrangements, and orienting group members are important factors in a group's effectiveness. The community health nurse can help to foster cohesiveness of groups by making certain that the four basic needs of a group are met and that blocks to group cohesiveness are avoided.

An understanding of the three predictable phases of group development will help the community health nurse recognize the developmental stage of a particular group. These three phases are dependence, counterdependence, and interdependence, and each of these phases is discussed in this chapter.

Once a group has formed there are group roles to be fulfilled. The group leader has a responsibility to help the group achieve its stated goals. The style of leadership, the performance of role activities, and the techniques used to carry out the group's functions will affect the group's ability to achieve its purpose. Nine leader interventions are discussed in this chapter.

Group members have specific roles that serve one of two basic functions necessary for a viable group. These roles are related to task roles and group maintenance roles. Task-related roles fall into two categories: process roles and content roles. Group maintenance roles are behaviors that promote a climate of cohesiveness and effective working relationships among group members. Dysfunctional roles hinder the group from reaching its goals and cannot be ignored.

Group problems that arise must be dealt with and resolved. Interpersonal conflict, dominance, and nonparticipation are common problems that group leaders and members must handle. At times the group leader and members must deal with emotional expressions such as crying or hostility. Each reaction must be handled in a supportive manner considering the individual's needs and the needs of the group. Leader responses should facilitate group process and outcomes.

Termination is an important phase in the life of a small group. Members should be prepared for the eventual termination of the group, and criteria for termination should be established. The group leader can facilitate the termination process by identifying criteria for termination at the onset of the group. While the group is occurring, the leader assists group members in working through their mixed feelings of loss, grief, or success or failure of the group goals as the group terminates.

Group evaluation includes assessing the ongoing group interaction (process measurement) as well as the effectiveness of the group (outcome measurement). The evaluation process should involve both the leader and group members. Process evaluation can be accomplished by periodic self-evaluation or by an outside observer. Outcome evaluation can be measured by determining how effective the group was in achieving its goal.

Working with populations (aggregates) can be compared with small-group work. A population group, in contrast to a small group, is a loose collection of people who have a quality or characteristic in common such as age, vunerability, or disease entity. The group usually arises out of some special need shared by a collection of people. Approaches on the part of the community health nurse in working with populations differ from those used in working with small groups. When working with populations the members do not necessarily have face to face contact and assessment and diagnosis of needs involve different strategies which may include interviewing, epidemiological surveys, examination of existing data, and conducting a collaborative needs assessment. The nursing process is presented as a tool for assessing, planning, implementing, and evaluating small group and population level intervention.

Teaching Strategies

A. Classroom Strategies

1. Use the Activities to Promote Critical Thinking in the text (Chapter 10) to generate discussion of phases of group development, comparison of a socialization group and a social group and/or an analysis of group member roles.

2. Assign seven to ten students to serve as a group. Have the group plan a group activity, assigning a specific maintenance or task role to each student in the group. Two or three additional students should be assigned the task of nonparticipating observer/recorder. The task of the group will be to plan an activity for National Nurses' Week or to choose a gift for the class to leave to the school. The goal for the group members will be to arrive at a consensus. Following the group process exercise the observers should report their observations of who they identified as acting in a specific role, and how the group worked to resolve conflict. Follow with a class discussion of the group dynamics led by the faculty member.

B. Clinical Laboratory Strategies

1. Assign individual students to observe a functioning group (not social) within the community and record their observations of the group process. Possible groups might include a weight management group, a faculty or agency planning meeting, or a self-help group at a local church or service organization.

2. Have the students develop a plan for initiating a task-oriented group or learning group within their clinical laboratory practice setting.

Evaluation Strategies

A. Multiple Choice Questions

1. Which of the following is an example of a learning group?
    a. An Alcoholics Anonymous meeting
    b. A group of refugees adapting to a new culture
    c. A childbirth education class
    d. A group of senior citizens planning a health fair

2. Which of the following is an example of a task-oriented group?
    a. An Alcoholics Anonymous meeting
    b. A group of refugees adapting to a new culture
    c. A childbirth education class
    d. A group of senior citizens planning a health fair

3. Which of the following is an example of a group formed primarily for support?
    a. A water aerobics class
    b. An Alateen meeting
    c. A prenatal clinic planning group
    d. A group of prisoners meeting prior to release

4. Which of the following factors can block group cohesiveness?
    a. Open membership
    b. Informal group norms
    c. Formation of task-specific and time- limited subgroups
    d. Stable communication channels

5. Group members perform specific roles within the group. What function is performed by the gatekeeper?
    a. Helps to keep communication channels open
    b. Offers facts, expresses feelings, and gives opinions
    c. Asks for factual clarification
    d. Expresses standards for the group

B. True/False Questions

1. The goal of a learning group is for members to change behavior in some area of need.
   a. True
   b. False

2. Socialization groups promote healthy behaviors and prevent maladaptive coping patterns.
   a. True
   b. False

3. Task-oriented groups are formed to promote the health of people with emotional disturbances.
   a. True
   b. False

4. Small group development goes through developmental phases.
   a. True
   b. False

5. Group termination is insignificant and does not warrant attention by the group leader or members.
   a. True
   b. False

C. Essay Questions

1. What role do you usually assume in a group? Explain what activities demonstrate this and explain what motivates you to assume this role. Does this role use all of your skills? Could you assume others? Which ones? How would you carry out these roles? (Use any or all of these questions in the essay you develop for students.)

2. You are working with very young (under sixteen) teen parents. Suggest groups these teens may benefit from. Is there one in your community? If not what would you plan. If so, how could you improve the services?

D. Individual or Group Projects

1. Use the Clinical Laboratory Strategies #1 or #2 and adapt the activities to become an individual or group activity.

2. If you belong to any of the types of groups discussed in this chapter choose one and observe the roles assumed by the group members. Describe the task related and maintenance related roles observed.

11

Using the Nursing Process to Promote the Health of Aggregates

Learning Objectives

- Describe each of the nursing process components as they apply to community health nursing.
- Identify data sources for assessing aggregate health.
- Formulate nursing diagnoses for aggregates.
- Develop a plan, including measurable goals and objectives, for addressing an identified aggregate health need.
- Describe the process of evaluating aggregate health interventions.
- Discuss characteristics of the nursing process affecting nursing practice with the community as client.

Key Terms

- Assessment
- Data base
- Evaluation
- Goals
- Implementation
- Interaction
- Needs
- Nursing Diagnosis
- Nursing Process
- Objectives
- Planning
- Setting Priorities

Chapter Summary

The nursing process is a systematic, purposeful set of nursing actions that includes assessment, diagnosis, planning, implementation and evaluation. All of these depend on a sixth component -interaction. For community health nursing in particular, the nurse-client interaction is an essential first consideration. Use of the nursing process as a tool provides nurses with three important capabilities: problem solving, managing nursing actions, and improving community health nursing practice.

Interaction is an important component of the nursing process. Interaction is a reciprocal and dynamic exchange between the nurse and the client and relies on mutual agreement and cooperation in order to succeed. Interaction at the community level focuses mainly on groups. Each person in the group is influenced by the others' behavior. Community health nursing interaction, therefore, is more complicated and complex than interaction between only two individuals. The success of all of the steps of the nursing process depends upon the quality of the nurse-client interaction.

Assessment is a means of determining client needs. It involves observing and judging the importance of all relevant signs, symptoms, or data. It has two steps: collecting and evaluating information about clients' health status in order to discover existing or potential needs as a basis for planning future action. There are two sources of data: primary, or information taken directly from the client, and secondary, or information coming from other persons, agencies, records, or reports. Data collection requires skillful observation, interviewing, listening, and direct examination. Data analysis and interpretation involves organizing the collected data in such a way that inferences or conclusions can be made and tested. Data can be categorized as physical, mental, social, or environmental, with each category examined for its particular significance. From this the nurse makes conclusions based on the data and validates these assumptions by including the clients in data interpretation.

Diagnosis, the next step in the nursing process, means that the nurse reaches a conclusion drawn from interpretation of collected data. In community health nursing the diagnosis focuses on a wellness response or a deficit response on the part of clients. Nurses do not limit their focus to problems; they look for evidence that may influence the clients' level of wellness, encompassing the whole length of the health-illness continuum.

Planning is a logical, methodical process of designing an orderly, detailed program of action to accomplish specific goals and objectives. Priority ranking must be done in situations involving multiple problems. Needs can be organized into categories, such as immediate, intermediate, and long-range. After establishing goals, the nurse establishes goals and objectives, and then writes an action plan. The action plan is designed to help the client achieve the objectives. A detailed example of how to record a nursing care plan is included on text pages 249-250.

Implementation involves putting the plan into action and seeing it through to completion in collaboration with the client. The nurse applies appropriate theories, provides a facilitative environment, assesses the client's readiness for service, carries out the plan or a modified version of it, and documents the progress of the implementation phase by process evaluation.

Evaluation is the final component of the nursing process and measures and judges the effectiveness of goal attainment. True evaluation uses standards that are the goals set with the client. The criteria that can be used to evaluate the goals are the specific objectives that were used as the stepping stones to each goal. Evaluation is the final component but not the end step in the nursing process. It is the beginning of the cyclical phase that establishes a continuation of interactions between the nurse and the client. Evaluating the quality of services, of program, and of nurse performance is receiving increased attention as the health care system is undergoing massive changes to become more cost efficient while providing effective services.

Certain characteristics within the nursing process are especially important for the community health nurse to emphasize. First is the deliberative nature of the nursing process. It is purposeful, rational, and well thought out acquiring sound judgement based on adequate information. It is adaptable, enabling the community health nurse to be flexible in meeting aggregate health needs. The nursing process is cyclical with the five steps repeated over and over as the nurse and client aggregate interact. It is client focused used expressly for addressing the health of populations. It is interactive wherein the nurse and clients engage in ongoing interpersonal communication. Finally, the nursing process is need-oriented, used by the nurse to anticipate clients' needs and prevent problems.

Teaching Strategies

A. Classroom Strategies

1. Ask a community health nurse (public health, school, agency) to discuss with the class a community health problem in which the nursing process was utilized to resolve the problem. Ask the nurse to discuss which of the methods of data collection on text pages 244-246 were used.
2. Have students compare and contrast how the nursing process is used in a variety of settings where well and ill clients are served.

B. Clinical Laboratory Strategies

1. Ask students to analyze data and develop a diagnosis and nursing care plan based on the community assessment they have been assigned as a clinical project.
2. Ask students to discuss how they will carry out the evaluation step of their plan of action based on their community assessment.

Evaluation Strategies

A. Multiple Choice Questions

1. Five major components of the nursing process are assessment, diagnosis, planning, implementation, and evaluation. These all depend on a sixth major component, which is
   a. client interaction.
   b. helping clients help themselves.
   c. an act of appraisal.
   d. data collection.

2. In community health, nurses do not limit their focus to problems. Community health nurses consider the client as a/an
   a. aggregate.
   b. broad diagnosis.
   c. total person.
   d. consultant.

3. Assessment involves
   a. collecting data.
   b. drawing conclusions.
   c. setting priorities.
   d. establishing goals.

4. Needs must be translated into which of the following to give direction and meaning to the nursing care plan?
   a. Implementation.
   b. Goals.
   c. Activities.
   d. Purposes.

5. A primary data source includes
   a. family members
   b. the client.
   c. research reports.
   d. health team members.

B. True/False Questions

1. The nursing process is deliberate and carefully thought out.
   a. True
   b. False

2. The data collection process in the nursing process focuses on one source of data.
   a. True
   b. False

3. Nursing diagnoses stay stable and unchanged during the time of caregiving to clients.
   a. True
   b. False

4. The nursing process is cyclical and the steps keep repeating over and over.
   a. True
   b. False

5. Evaluation requires specific standards and criteria by which to judge outcomes of care.
   a. True
   b. False

C. Essay Questions

1. Provide students with a community health case study. Ask them to outline steps in the nursing process and identify appropriate nursing activities to promote client wellness.

2. Describe how you would complete the assessment phase of the nursing process with an individual client and an aggregate client. Would there be a difference? Why or why not?

D. Individual or Group Projects

1. Assess the quality assurance system of a clinical agency with which you are familiar. Use the five points listed on p. 252 in the text, Chapter 11 to guide your assessment.

2. Using the same case study in essay #1, have students make a list of data sources and information needed before forming a diagnosis and beginning the planning phase.

12 Epidemiological Assessment of Community Health Status

Learning Objectives

- Explain the host, agent, and environment model.
- Describe theories of causality in health and illness.
- Define immunity and explain passive, active, cross, and herd immunity.
- Explain how epidemiologists determine populations at risk.
- Explain the four stages of a disease or health condition.
- List the major sources of epidemiological information.
- Distinguish between incidence and prevalence in health and illness states.
- Use epidemiologic methods to describe an aggregate's health.
- Distinguish between types of epidemiologic studies useful for researching aggregate health.

Key Terms

- Agent
- Analytic epidemiology
- Causality
- Cohort
- Descriptive epidemiology
- Epidemiology
- Experimental epidemiology
- Host
- Immunity
- Incidence
- Morbidity rate
- Mortality rate
- Prevalence
- Prospective study
- Rates
- Retrospective study
- Risk

Chapter Summary

Epidemiology is defined in this chapter as "the study of the distribution and determinants of health, disease, and injuries in human populations." The primary goal of epidemiology is to find the causes of health problems and identify solutions to prevent disease and improve the health of the entire population. Community health nurses use epidemiology as a frame of reference for assessing the health of population groups and for improving clinical practice.

The term epidemiology is derived from the Greek words epi (upon) demos (the people) and logos (knowledge). The historical background of epidemiology can be traced to Hippocrates, who is often referred to as the first epidemiologist. Modern epidemiology, however, did not come into existence until the late nineteenth century.

Early epidemiology was concerned with the study of epidemics of infectious disease. Plague spread through Europe and England in 1348 and killed millions of people over many years. Bubonic and pneumonic plague have appeared and reappeared at times. As the great epidemic diseases declined other diseases were focused on by epidemiologists such as diptheria, typhoid, tuberculosis, dysentery, and syphilis. Nursing epidemiologic roots can be traced back to Florence Nightingale's detailed records on health conditions among the military in the Crimean War. This represented one of the first descriptive studies of the distribution and determinants of disease in a population. She used statistical data along with her records to bring about environmental changes. Through the years, community health nurses have continued to work to improve the environment.

Several early theories of disease causation are described in this chapter. Sydenham's miasma theory dominated early thought. Noxious vapors associated with the decay of organic matter were thought to cause disease. Later the contagion theory was developed. Although the thinking behind these theories was faulty, the resulting preventive measures had positive effects. As ideas of disease causation changed, the concept of multiple causation emerged. This model, referred to as the "web of causation," attempts to identify all of the possible influences on the health and illness process.

The tripartite model of the interaction among the susceptible host, causal agent, and environment has been used by epidemiologists to study disease. The major challenge of epidemiologic studies is to identify causal relationships in disease or health conditions.

The concept of immunity and the four types that are important to community health are explored. The four types are passive, active, cross, and herd immunity. The probability that a disease or health problem will occur is known as the risk. Epidemiologist study populations at risk and measure their risk potential.

Epidemiologic investigators draw data from three major sources of information: 1) existing data from the census bureau and reportable disease statistics, 2) informal investigations and inquiry and 3) carefully designed scientific studies. The natural history or progression of a disease or condition occurs in four stages: susceptibility, exposure, onset, and culmination. The stages are discussed on pages 266-267. New epidemiologic models of wellness are being developed and are organized around attributes that influence health. Several societal changes such as an increased aging population, global economy and technical developments are driving these new approaches.

Two basic methods of investigation for epidemiologic studies are observation and experimentation. Observational studies can be either descriptive studies, which seek to describe health-related conditions as they naturally occur, and analytic studies, which look for causal factors.

The goal of a descriptive study is to identify patterns of occurrence. Counts, rates and other forms of statistical analysis are used. Counts are the simplest way to present data and may be expressed as ratios or proportions. The most important rates for the community health nurse to understand include prevalence rates, period prevalence rates, and incidence rates. The significance of these rates and formulas for calculating them are on pages 273-274 in the text. Additional rates used to make comparisons among populations are mortality rates, infant mortality rates, and case fatality rates.

Analytic studies constitute the second type of observational epidemiologic study. This form of study differs from a descriptive study only in that an attempt is made to determine causal factors.

In experimental studies the factors suspected of causing a particular health condition are actually controlled or changed by the investigator. The investigator compares the group with the exposure factor against a matched group without the exposure factor. A community trial is a type of experimental study done at the community level..

The investigation process of an epidemiologic study involves seven steps: 1) identify the problem, 2) review the literature, 3) design the study, 4) collect the data, 5) analyze the findings, 6) develop conclusions and applications, and 7) disseminate the findings. Community health nurses are constantly confronted with threats to the community's health and well-being, and these concerns are potential areas of study.

Teaching Strategies

A. Classroom Strategies

1. Select a topic or have the class identify a problem or concern that is a threat to the health and well-being of their community, such as drug abuse, teenage pregnancies, high school dropout rates, or sexually transmitted diseases. Guide the class through the seven steps of the epidemiologic investigative process. Demonstrate how the multiple causation theory can be used as a conceptual model for the study developed by the class.

2. Invite a nurse-epidemiologist from a local public health agency to speak to the class about his/her role.

B. Clinical Laboratory Strategies

1. Assign to students clients needing epidemiologic follow-up (such as TB or Salmonella investigations) and have them share their experiences with other students during a clinical conference.

2. Encourage students to participate in epidemiological studies being conducted by community agencies as part of their clinical laboratory experience. Share the experience during a clinical laboratory conference.

Evaluation Strategies

A. Multiple Choice Questions

1. The tripartite epidemiological model includes
   a. health, illness, and injuries.
   b. incidence, prevalence, and case fatality.
   c. host, agent, and environment.
   d. immunity, causation, and risk.

2. Epidemiologic investigations focus on
   a. communicable diseases.
   b. skin conditions in the workplace.
   c. causes of dermatological illnesses.
   d. causation of disease and injury.

3. A case-control study is an observational study that
   a. describes patterns of occurrence of illness and injury in a population.
   b. compares persons with a health-illness condition and persons without the condition.
   c. investigates the development of a health-illness condition over a long period of time.
   d. studies a cohort and evaluates variables associated with the disease or injury.

4. A community trial is
   a. an inexpensive type of analytic study.
   b. a type of experimental study done at the community level.
   c. a study that gathers volunteers for the experimental group.
   d. a way to locate health problems in a variety of communities.

5. The concept of causality refers to
   a. the relationship between a cause and its effect.
   b. all the possible influences on the health and illness processes.
   c. the host's ability to resist infectious disease-causing agents.
   d. the chances that a disease or health problem will occur.

B. True/False Questions

1. Epidemiology is defined as the study of distribution and determinants of health, disease, and injuries in populations.
   a. True
   b. False

2. Incidence refers to all people with a health condition existing in a given population at a given point in time.
   a. True
   b. False

3. Epidemiologic studies are a form of research.
   a. True
   b. False

4. Natural passive immunity occurs through maternal antibody transfer.
   a. True
   b. False

5. Naturally acquired active immunity comes through vaccine inoculation.
   a. True
   b. False

C. Essay Questions

1. Using the seven steps of the epidemiologic process, follow a specific community health illness or injury condition through the steps. Identify how a study on the selected topic could be conducted locally with the resources known to be available.

2. Identify a community health issue of importance to you. What studies do you feel need to be conducted on this topic? How could you go about beginning to research this issue. What agencies might you involve?

D. Individual or Group Projects

1. Assign student(s) to visit the local health department to observe how data is obtained, recorded, and analyzed. Have the student(s) report observations to the clinical laboratory group or classmates.

2. Using a research article that includes an epidemiologic study, have students design a similar investigation in their own community. Needed modifications and changes in the design should be included. This is intended to be a paper and pencil exercise but may develop into an actual study if the opportunity presents itself.

Communication and Collaboration in Community Health

13

Learning Objectives

- Identify the seven parts of the communication process.
- Describe four barriers to effective communication in community health and how to deal with them.
- Explain three sets of skills necessary for effective communication in community health nursing.
- Discuss four techniques for enhancing group decision making.
- Describe five characteristics of collaboration in community health.
- Identify four features of community health contracting.
- Develop an aggregate level contact in community health.

Key Terms

- Active listening
- Brainstorming
- Channel
- Collaboration
- Communication
- Contracting
- Decoding
- Delphi technique
- Electronic meetings
- Empathy
- Encoding
- Feedback loop
- Formal contracting
- Informal contracting
- Message
- Nominal group technique
- Nonverbal messages
- Receiver
- Sender
- Verbal messages

Chapter Summary

Communication and collaboration form the basis for effective working relationships of community health nurses. Communicating with aggregates to prevent illness and protect and promote health takes special skills and tools. This chapter examines these tools and how the community health nurse develops and integrates them into community health nursing practice.

The communication process engages in an exchange that is both understood and meaningful. The process has seven parts that need to work together to have meaning. They are: 1) the message, 2) a sender, 3) a receiver, 4) encoding, 5), a channel, 6) decoding, and 7) a feedback loop. Each part is described in this chapter.

There are barriers to effective communication. Four pose particular problems: sender and receivers selective perception; language barriers from slang, regional or foreign/cultural differences; filtering or manipulating information by the sender; and an emotional state that may cloud the perception of the message.

Three sets of communication skills, sending skills, receiving skills, and interpersonal skills are essential for successful development of an effective nurse-client relationship. In order to communicate effectively, it is essential that community health nurses, as senders of messages, have awareness of their own personal feelings and motives and are also aware that the wants and needs of receivers will influence receivers' perceptions of the message sent.

Messages may be sent verbally or nonverbally. Nearly two-thirds of all messages are transmitted nonverbally. Nonverbal messages are sent through body language, facial expressions, gestures, and tone of voice. Some basic rules for effective communication are to "keep the message honest and uncomplicated; use as few words as possible to state it, and ask for reactions (feedback) to make certain that it is understood".

Receiving skills are as important to communication as sending skills. The community health nurse needs to listen actively, to use reflective questions to clarify and show interest, and to observe behavior. Previous experiences, culture, and participant relationship strongly influence the meaning and understanding attached to messages.

Community health nursing requires interpersonal skills in addition to effective communication skills. The interpersonal skills of showing respect, empathizing, and developing trust build on sending and receiving skills but go beyond the mere exchange of messages. An attitude of respect conveys to clients that they are important and have dignity and worth. Empathy tells clients that the nurse shares their concerns. Trust generates trust and develops through an open and honest approach with clients.

Community health nurses are actively involved in group decision making. Four functions are of particular relevance to group decision-making. First, community group members share information. Secondly, they present diverse views and generate alternatives to the problem-solving process. Thirdly, group member's thinking is influenced and perspectives are broadened thus improving the quality of the group's decisions. Finally, time pressure and desire for completion help the group progress toward consensus and/or resolution. There are several useful techniques for exhausting group decision-making. They are brainstorming, nominal group technique, Delphi technique, and electronic meetings. Each method is described in this chapter.

Collaboration for community health nurses means purposeful interactions between nurses, clients, and other community members based on mutual participation and joint effort. Collaboration has a goal to benefit the public's health. There are four characteristics that distinguish collaboration from other types of interaction: shared goals, mutual participation, maximized resources, and clear responsibilities. Once the purpose for collaborating has been accomplished, the group can be terminated. Because the relationship is bound by time, the structure involves a beginning phase of establishing the team, a middle or working phase, and a termination phase as the relationship ends. Most clients have had limited experience collaborating with health personnel, especially clients from poverty areas, from different cultural backgrounds, or with little or no formal education. They may need extensive encouragement to participate actively. The nurse's own view of collaboration will also influence the degree of client participation.

Community health nurses often use contracting as a technique to assist clients to assume responsibility for their own health and achieve self-care. The concept of contracting negotiates a working agreement between two or more parties and has four distinct features: partnership, commitment, format, and negotiation. The contracting process is viewed as a partnership between the nurse and the client. Both should participate in developing the agreement. Every contract implies a commitment to fulfill the purpose of the agreement. A third feature is format. The contract provides a framework for the nurse-client relationship. It should spell out exactly what must be done, who is to do it, and within what time frame it is to be accomplished. Negotiation involves give-and-take, with the participants making compromises about the terms of the contract.

Contracting has some potential problems if it places a client under stress, impedes trust, or negatively influences the relationship. The advantages however are many; it involves clients in promoting their own health; motivates clients to perform necessary tasks; focuses on clients' unique needs; increases the possibility of achieving health goals identified by collaborating team members; enhances all team members' problem-solving skills; fosters client participation in the decision-making process; promotes clients' autonomy and self-esteem as they learn self-care; and makes nursing services more efficient and cost effective.

The steps of contracting may vary in sequence or may overlap. The phases are 1) exploration of needs, 2) establishment of goals, 3) exploration of resources, 4) development of a plan, 5) division of responsibility, 6) agreement on time frame, 7) evaluation, and 8) renegotiation or termination. Figure 13.4, p. 296 in the text depicts the concept and process of contracting.

The contracting process may be conducted on a formal or informal level. On a formal level, a written contract is drawn up. In other cases an informal verbal agreement is sufficient. The selection of the contracting level depends on the skill of the nurse, readiness of the client and demands of the situation.

Teaching Strategies

A. Classroom Strategies

1. Bring samples of formal contracts that have been used by a community health nurse, or prepare several samples of your own. Ask students to review the contracts and then evaluate the terms spelled out in the agreements.

2. Ask for student volunteers to role-play a nurse-client (family) situation. One of the student volunteers should be selected by the group to play the role of a community health nurse. The remaining students should decide which family member roles they want to act out. The community health nurse's assignment will be to negotiate an informal contract with the family. The contract could be related to one of the following issues: weight management, compliance with a medical regime, or hygiene practices. The class as a whole will then critique the role-playing situation in relation to the contracting process and the communication skills and tools used.

B. Clinical Laboratory Strategies

1. Assign the students to observe a community health nurse in a practice setting. Have the students identify the communication skills and the collaborative process used. Each student should record their analysis of the situation in a journal. (This may be part of an observational experience to meet some other clinical laboratory objectives.)

2. Suggest that students select a client from their clinical laboratory practice setting and negotiate a formal or informal contract. This exercise may be simulated or, if appropriate, actually carried out. Ask students to record in a journal the events that took place during the contracting process.

Evaluation Strategies

A. Multiple Choice Questions

1. The communication process has seven parts. An important one is
    a. a feedback loop.
    b. setting responsibilities.
    c. being goal-directed.
    d. a time-limit.

2. Barriers to effective communication as mentioned in this chapter include
    a. clients' use of medical terminology.
    b. selective perception on the part of the nurse or client.
    c. sharing complete and accurate information.
    d. taking people's differences into account during communication.

3. Collaboration is distinguished from other types of interaction by
    a. always including a client within the team.
    b. lengthening the time needed to meet goals.
    c. flexible boundaries and responsibilities.
    d. shared goals and mutual participation.

4. The group decision-making technique of brainstorming includes
    a. sharing all ideas and suggestions before discussion begins.
    b. discussion after the generation of each idea.
    c. ongoing constructive criticism offered by the leader.
    d. alternating ideas and suggestions with feedback and criticism.

5. Benefits of contracting with clients include
    a. decreasing client stress.
    b. contributing to a trusting nurse-client relationship.
    c. reducing client visit time by over fifty percent.
    d. fostering client participation in the decision-making process.

B. True/False Questions

1. Nearly one-third of all messages are transmitted nonverbally.
    a. True
    b. False

2. Sending skills are more important than receiving skills.
   a. True
   b. False

3. When the sender manipulates information he/she creates a barrier to effective communication.
   a. True
   b. False

4. The Delphi Technique is a group decision making activity.
   a. True
   b. False

5. A written grant proposal is an example of an informal contract.
   a. True
   b. False

C. Essay Questions

1. Select a group decision making technique and identify how this technique will help solve the following two problems: 1) services being offered to prenatal clients in your agency are not well attended, and 2) agency employees are unhappy about the way vacation dates are determined.

2. Provide an example of a formal contract and suggest how the community health nurse could present the idea in the following examples: 1) a family has a history of obesity and wants to change this pattern, 2) a group of seniors at a local senior center would like a community health nurse to provide health information classes on a regular basis, 3) your agency and a pharmaceutical company are collaborating on testing a new ostomy product on selected clients.

D. Individual or Group Projects

1. Collect samples of contracts used in a variety of settings with different groups of clients. Compare and contrast the contracts. Select parts of each contract that appeal to you the most in order to develop model contracts for future use.

2. With a group of peers, participate in a variety of role-playing scenarios which demonstrate core communication skills, barriers to effective communication, and collaboration. "Contract" with the faculty member to demonstrate these techniques as part of your course grade.

Educational Interventions to Promote Community Health

14

Learning Objectives

- Examine the community health nurse's role as teacher in promoting health, and preventing or postponing morbidity.
- Choose selected learning theories that are applicable to an individual, family, or aggregate client.
- Select teaching methods and materials that facilitate learning for clients at different development levels.
- Develop teaching plans focusing on primary, secondary, and tertiary levels of prevention for clients of all ages.
- Identify teaching strategies the nurse can use when encountering the "hard to help" client.
- Locate appropriate audio-visual and printed material resources to enhance client teaching.

Key Terms

- Accommodation (Piaget)
- Adaptation (Piaget)
- Affective domain
- Anticipatory guidance
- Assimilation (Piaget)
- Cognitive domain
- Deductive
- Gestalt-field
- Learning
- Levels of prevention
- Operant conditioning
- Operationalize
- Primary prevention
- Psychomotor domain
- Secondary prevention
- Teaching

Chapter Summary

The educator role of the nurse is basic to community health nursing. Keeping clients healthy through teaching and/or changing behaviors that will improve the quality and quantity of the client's life are the nurse's goals. In order to accomplish these goals the nurse must know about the nature and domains of learning and be familiar with various learning theories. From a practical point of view, the nurse's effectiveness as an educator will be enhanced by having knowledge of teaching-learning principles, the teaching process, and methods and materials to use when teaching.

The nurse as a teacher seeks to transmit information in such a way that the learner (client) understands and some measurable change in behavior results. To achieve this change, learning theories are used. A learning theory is described as a "systematic and integrated outlook in regard to the nature of the process whereby people relate to their environments in such a way as to enhance their ability to use both themselves and their environments more effectively" (Biggs, 1992, p.3). Three categories of learning theories are discussed in this chapter. Behavioral focuses on behaviors that can be observed, measured, and changed through stimulus-response or conditioning. Cognitive focuses on the understanding of problems and situations and the ability to think, perceive, abstract, and generalize information through promoting their insights. Humanistic assumes that there is a natural tendency for people to learn and that learning flourishes in an encouraging environment. It is brought out in this chapter that the nurse may combine one or more learning theories and each nurse has a preferential style of teaching that may focus on one theory more than another.

Learning occurs in three domains: cognitive, affective, and psychomotor (Tables 14-1, 14-2, and 14-3, pages 305, 306, 307, and 310). The cognitive domain refers to learning that takes place intellectually and ranges from simple recall to complex evaluation, along six levels of learning. Affective learning involves a change of attitudes and values and this may be achieved at several levels of affective involvement from simple listening to adopting a new value. Psychomotor learning involves the acquisition of motor skills which includes being capable of the skill, developing a sensory image of the skill, and practicing the skill.

Effective teaching is the responsibility of the educator, but learning is the responsibility of the learner. Basic principles of teaching-learning (Table 14.5 p. 311) relate to client readiness, client perceptions, physical and emotional comfort within the educational setting, relevancy of the subject matter, client satisfaction, and reinforcement of the learning through application. The teaching method suggested in this chapter is similar to the nursing process in that it contains the following elements: interaction, assessment and diagnosis, goal setting, planning, teaching, and evaluation.

The teaching methods described in this chapter include lecture, discussion, demonstration, and role playing. A variety of teaching tools and materials are suggested to prepare the nurse to teach the individual, family, or group effectively. Some clients are "hard to help" and strategies are shared to enhance a challenging teaching situation.

Teaching Strategies

A. Classroom Strategies

1. Have students select and provide rationale for using a learning theory that is applicable to an individual, family, or aggregate for each of the following scenarios: A young mother in need of enhanced parenting skills; an intergenerational family of seven members who has a terminally ill member being cared for at home; and an aggregate of preschool aged children needing a class on personal hygiene.

2. Following your lecture on the seven teaching-learning principles, ask students to identify how they were used in the presentation.

3. Ask students to select teaching methods and materials that would be appropriate in the three scenarios presented in number 1.

B. Clinical Laboratory Strategies

1. Each student should select a teaching project to implement with a community group of their choice. Each student should submit a formal teaching plan which includes name of group, contact person, teaching topic, evidence of learner readiness, behavioral objectives, outline of content, methods and materials used (with rationale), and evaluation strategies.

2. Each student should present 10 minutes of the plan to their peers during a clinical conference. The peers should "behave" like the intended learners might. After the presentation, the other students and you should verbally critique the sample of teaching and give positive and negative feedback that will enhance the teaching with the intended learners.

3. Have the student implement the teaching plan with the intended learners and you in attendance. After the teaching session, give verbal and written feedback for student growth in the role of teacher.

Evaluation Strategies

A. Multiple Choice Questions

1. The following example demonstrates the knowledge level of cognitive learning. After attending the nurse's class on nutrition the client
   a. can name three foods high in iron.
   b. compares the nutrient value in food.
   c. eats well balanced meals.
   d. adapts recipes to be low in fat.

2. The following example demonstrates the application level of cognitive learning. After attending the nurse's class on nutrition the client
   a. can name three foods high in iron.
   b. compares the nutrient value in food.
   c. eats well balanced meals.
   d. adapts recipes to be low in fat.

3. Behavioral theory focuses on
   a. meeting a hierarchy of needs.
   b. the understanding of the problem.
   c. a person's natural tendency to learn.
   d. changes in response to a stimulus.

4. The teaching process has sequential steps similar to
   a. affective learning.
   b. cognitive theory.
   c. the nursing process.
   d. teaching-learning principles.

5. Cognitive learning is sequential. Of the following examples, which is in the correct progressive order?
   a. Application, knowledge, synthesis
   b. Comprehension, analysis, evaluation
   c. Analysis, application, evaluation
   d. Synthesis, comprehension, knowledge

B. True/False Questions

1. The goal of teaching is the sharing of information.
    a. True
    b. False

2. The humanistic theory of learning assumes that learning flourishes in an encouraging environment.
    a. True
    b. False

3. Knowledge is the highest level of cognitive learning and involves recall.
    a. True
    b. False

4. An example of a psychomotor skill in community health is infant bathing.
    a. True
    b. False

5. Client readiness for learning is affected by maturation.
    a. True
    b. False

C. Essay Questions

1. Select one topic to teach (nutrition, safety, or exercise, etc.) and adapt it to preschoolers and senior citizens. Identify the appropriate learning objectives, methods and materials, and evaluation methods for each group. Include the rationale for the differences you select.

2. Write a behavioral objective at each of the 6 levels of cognitive learning for a selected topic.

D. Individual or Group Projects

1. Have small groups of students develop behavioral objectives at different levels of cognitive learning for several different topics. Write them for all to see. Have the students critique them for measurability and appropriateness.

2. Observe a community health nurse teaching a group of clients and critique his/her effectiveness. What suggestions might you give the nurse? What behaviors might you like to incorporate into your own teaching style?

Community Crisis: Prevention and Intervention

15

Learning Objectives

- Define crisis.
- Describe the phases of a crisis.
- Explain the difference between developmental crisis and situational crisis and give several examples of each.
- Plan strategies to prevent situational crisis and developmental crisis at each level of prevention.
- Describe the role of a community heath nurse in crisis intervention during each phase of the crisis.

Key Terms

- Bargaining
- Coping
- Crisis
- Crisis Theory

- Developmental crisis
- Post-crisis Phase
- Pre-crisis Phase
- Situational crisis

Chapter Summary

A crisis is an event that comes with or without warning and disturbs the equilibrium of a person, group, or community. Crisis can bring a turning point to people's lives that creates a growth situation or an inclination to stress and disease. *Crisis theory* is the body of knowledge which explains why people respond in certain ways during crises. Crisis theory also helps us to understand the predictable phases of response individuals, groups, and communities go through before, during, and after a crisis.

The dynamics of crisis can be understood by considering how people, as living systems, tend to behave. Human beings (generally unconsciously) try to maintain equilibrium within themselves and in their relations with others. When internal or external forces upset this equilibrium, people try to cope by using their usual problem-solving methods. Tension occurs and builds when a person is unable to resolve the situation. Ideally people seek and receive outside help and find new ways to solve the problem. With others, the problem remains unresolved, leading to tragic circumstances such as family disruption, psychiatric breakdowns, or even death.

Crisis phases are predictable and sequential which allows the community caregiver to give optimum help at the right time. The pre-crisis phase, the time before a crisis occurs, is when primary prevention activities take place. Depending on the type of crisis, the pre-crisis phase may not allow for any preparation or prevention, such as with a derailed train. When a river's water begins to rise to flood stage, a community may have sufficient time to prepare and be safe.

During the crisis phase those involved are in a state of shock, are very vulnerable to suggestions, and may respond in a variety of ways. Their response should be considered normal and managed symptomatically. During the post-crisis phase, healing and recovery is achieved through expert assistance, as people attempt to regain equilibrium. It is during this phase that the help received by the people or community allows the crisis to be a growth experience. Without the assistance, the crisis may never be resolved.

There are two types of crises, developmental and situational. Developmental crises occur at transition points in normal growth and development. This type of crisis usually has a gradual onset and can be anticipated. Examples of a developmental crisis are the high school graduation of a family member or the expansion of housing into the suburbs. A situational crisis is unexpected and externally imposed, most frequently with a sudden onset and little or no time to prepare. Examples of situational rises include accidents, natural disasters, and unemployment. At times people experience multiple crises. The effects of multiple crises may be too much for many people to manage with their usual coping strategies. Help from the community health nurse and others is much needed and desired.

To intervene in a crisis, the nurse can practice primary, secondary, and tertiary prevention. Primary prevention involves preventing the crisis from occurring in the first place. This can often be achieved by meeting basic needs. When basic needs, such as safe working conditions are provided, the population is less vulnerable to physical, mental, or psychosocial problems. Through anticipatory guidance, the nurse can help clients plan for the future so that they can help themselves when and if a crisis arises. Secondary prevention involves early detection and treatment to reduce the intensity and duration of the crisis. The nurse can help the individual, family or community minimize the effects of the crisis which allows for a fuller recovery in the post-crisis phase. Tertiary prevention strives to reduce the amount and degree of disability or damage as a result of a crisis. It can go beyond rehabilitation to include helping the client reduce the risk of future crises.

The two major methods for crisis intervention are the generic and individual approaches. The generic approach deals with a single type of crisis, such as an infant death, and often works with groups of people involved in the same type of crisis. The individual approach is used when clients need additional therapy. Crisis intervention begins with assessment of the situation, followed by planning a therapeutic intervention, and implementation by building on the strengths and self-care ability of the clients. Crisis intervention concludes with resolution and anticipatory planning to avert possible future crises.

Teaching Strategies

A. Classroom Strategies

1. Discuss the role that the mass media play in a national crisis, such as the Oklahoma City bombing, or a recent natural disaster.

2. Select a recent crisis of local, regional or national proportion, that all students are familiar with and discuss 1) the category of crisis, 2) role of the nurse at the primary, secondary, and tertiary levels, and 3) the crisis intervention steps the nurse could take.

3. Invite a representative of the local chapter of the American Red Cross to discuss their disaster response capabilities and the role of a volunteer disaster nurse.

B. Clinical Laboratory Strategies

1. In the community assessment that the students conduct, have them try to identify a community crisis that has occurred in the past. How was the crisis managed and resolved? What were the outcomes?

2. After completing a community assessment, have students determine what potential crisis this community may experience, such as a factory fire, flooding,

or an outbreak of a communicable disease. Have the students prepare a plan to prevent such a crisis.

3. Ask each student to develop a disaster preparedness plan with each assigned family. Include such items as fire exit plans, storage of poisons, emergency phone numbers, and so forth.

Evaluation Strategies

A. Multiple Choice Questions

1. A crisis is defined as
   a. a way of life for some families.
   b. an uncomfortable but not risky situation.
   c. a temporary disequilibrium in life.
   d. an avoidable situation.

2. A developmental crisis is
   a. an externally imposed accident.
   b. precipitated by a life transition.
   c. sudden in onset and unexpected.
   d. precipitated by a hazardous event.

3. Primary crisis prevention involves
   a. meeting basic needs through anticipatory guidance.
   b. early detection and response to the crisis.
   c. rehabilitation and restoration of lives.
   d. the work of official agencies during the crisis.

4. The community health nurse teaches two young parents what growth and developmental changes to expect in their 3 month old child in the next 6 months. These activities are conducted at which phase of a crisis?
   a. Pre-crisis
   b. Crisis
   c. Post-crisis
   d. Situational crisis

5. The goal of crisis intervention is to
   a. prevent the crisis altogether.
   b. involve as many people as possible in the resolution.
   c. triage clients during the post-crisis phase.
   d. reestablish equilibrium to the lives of those involved.

B. True/False Questions

1. Developmental crises are the expected transitional events in a person's life.
   a. True
   b. False

2. Community health nurses do not intervene in crises at the pre-crisis phase.
   a. True
   b. False

3. A personal family situation is not considered a crisis.
   a. True
   b. False

4. The early part of the crisis phase is when the client first encounters the crisis situation.
   a. True
   b. False

5. In the late crisis phase, clients begin to display shock.
   a. True
   b. False

C. Essay Questions

1. One of your clients, the Smyth family, is planning a large family reunion with over 100 anticipated guests. Make several suggestions that will help your clients experience this event with the least amount of stress.

2. You come upon a traffic accident in a rural part of your county. There are several injured people and two bystanders. Outline your actions as a community health nurse at this crisis event. Give your rationale for each action.

D. Individual or Group Projects

1. Use the situation in essay question number 2 and have the students work in small groups and outline the nurses' actions and rationale for each action.

2. Have each student survey his or her own home and develop a disaster preparedness plan.

Theoretical Bases for Promoting Family Health

16

Learning Objectives

- Analyze changing definitions of family.
- Discuss characteristics all families have in common.
- List the traditional and nontraditional units that make up families.
- Describe the functions of a family.
- Identify the developmental tasks of a family as it grows.
- Analyze the role of the community health nurse in promoting the health of the family unit.

Key Terms

- Blended family
- Cohabitating couples
- Commune family
- Commuter family
- Energy exchange
- Family
- Family culture
- Family functioning
- Family map
- Family structure
- Family system boundary
- Foster families
- Gangs
- Group-marriage family
- Group-network family
- Homeless family
- Intrarole functioning
- Kin-network
- Multigenerational family
- Nontraditional family
- Nuclear-dyad family
- Nuclear family
- Primary relationship
- Roles
- Single-adult family
- Single-parent family
- Traditional family

Chapter Summary

The family is the basic unit of service in community health nursing. Chapter 16 provides the student with an overview of the underlying theories, characteristics, functions, and tasks of the family. The community health nurses' effectiveness in working with families depends on understanding family theory and characteristics, in addition to the changing family structures of today. A growing body of research on families has provided a great deal of information about how families are structured and how they function.

Every family is unique and yet shares some universal characteristics with other families. Every family: 1) is a small social system, 2) has its own cultural values and rules, 3) has structure, 4) has certain basic functions, and 5) moves through stages in its life cycle. These five family universals provide the framework for looking at families in this chapter.

Families, as social systems set and maintain boundaries that unite them and preserve their autonomy while also differentiating them from others. Families are equilibrium-seeking and adaptive systems that strive to adjust to internal and external life changes. Families are goal directed and exist for the purpose of promoting their members' development.

A family has its own set of values and rules for operation and shares a culture. This family culture influences member beliefs and behaviors. These same values prescribe the types of roles that each member assumes, power distribution and decision-making patterns. Family structure can be categorized as either traditional or nontraditional (see Table 16-1, p. 351). The traditional structures are more inclusive than in years past and include nuclear families, couples without children, single-parent families, single-adult families, divorced families (50% of all marriages end in divorce, see Table 16-4, p. 360 for phases, emotional responses and transitional issues when families divorce), blended families (this group is also growing, see Table 16-5, p. 361 which describes phases, emotional responses and developmental issues), multigenerational families and kin networks. Nontraditional family structures incorporate many forms, some accepted by society and others not easily accepted. These variations include commune families, group marriages, group networks, unmarried single-parent families, and unmarried gay or straight couples living together with or without children, homeless families, foster families, and "gangs". These nontraditional families make up an increasing proportion of the United States population.

Every family has certain basic functions. Families give their members affection, emotional support, security, social and personal identity, and a sense of belonging. A stable family environment maintains the physical needs of its members. Families progress through predictable developmental stages (Table 16-3, p. 359). Families develop in two broad stages: a period of expansion when they add new members and roles and a period of contraction when members leave. Figure 16-4, p. 357 depicts Duvall's eight stages of the nuclear family life cycle and the relative percent of life time spent in each stage.

Teaching Strategies

A. Classroom Strategies

1. Discuss several popular television situation comedies or dramas. Ask students to identify the family structures depicted in these shows. Which are traditional and which are nontraditional (use Table 16-1, p. 352)? How well do these TV families fulfill the functions and tasks as depicted in Table 16-2, p. 355?

2. Suggest that students volunteer to describe their own family structure using the appropriate Tables from Chapter 16. Discuss the differences shared.

3. Throughout the course have students collect impressions of traditional and nontraditional family functioning from community health nurses practicing in a variety of settings. Compare and contrast the nurses' views.

B. Clinical Laboratory Strategies

1. Have each student assess assigned families in relation to being a traditional or nontraditional family. Share this information among peers. What percent are traditional families? What percent are nontraditional families? How many are nuclear families? Did any of the percentages surprise the students? Which percentages and why?

2. Have the students repeat the above exercise with their clients over the age of 65. Ask the older adults about the family structure they grew up in. Have the statistics changed using an older population? If so, what might be the reasons?

3. Each student selects a family he or she is providing care for and assesses them for their ability to meet family functions and tasks as outlined in Table 16-2, p. 355. Share the findings during a clinical laboratory conference.

Evaluation Strategies

A. Multiple Choice Questions

1. Which of the following best describes the most advanced definition of family?
    a. The family is who the client says it is
    b. Only persons who are related by a common inheritance
    c. Persons who are involved in the same social groups in a community
    d. Persons who live in close proximity to each other

2. Family system boundaries are best described as
    a. closed.
    b. semi-permeable.
    c. open.
    d. obstructed.

3. Family values determine
    a. family members' beliefs, thoughts, and feelings.
    b. alienation of family member from each other.
    c. physiological behaviors of family members.
    d. economic problems of a family.

4. In what way does a nuclear dyad differ from a nuclear family?
    a. The children in a nuclear dyad family are infants and not walking yet
    b. The children in a nuclear dyad family are of school age
    c. A nuclear dyad family is childless or the children are launched
    d. A nuclear dyad family is multigenerational

5. Which of the following is an example of a nontraditional family?
    a. A nuclear family
    b. A divorced family
    c. A commuter family
    d. A homeless family

B. True/False Questions

1. The definition of family is becoming broader and includes more nontraditional living arrangements.
    a. True
    b. False

2. In order for a group of people to be classified as a "family" there must be children.
    a. True
    b. False

3. The blended family has always been considered a traditional family.
    a. True
    b. False

4. A family functions for several reasons, one of which is to provide affection.
   a. True
   b. False

5. As a family reaches the teenage stage, its control function has more clearly defined limits.
   a. True
   b. False

C. Essay Questions

1. The Jones' have been married for six years. They have 4 children. Two (aged 16 and 13) are from Mrs. Jones first marriage, one (age 9) is from Mr. Jones first marriage, and their 3 year old is from their union. Using the family characteristics outlined in this chapter, describe the type of family and the appropriate stage-critical family developmental tasks you as a student community health nurse would include in a family assessment or in providing anticipatory guidance to this family.

2. "Gangs" are considered a nontraditional family. Identify how a community health nurse could work effectively with high risk youth at the primary, secondary or tertiary level of prevention to promote individual members' health.

D. Individual or Group Projects

1. Have each student keep a journal of their own family interactions during the duration of the course and note areas that could be worked on to have a healthier family life.

2. Select a family you are familiar with and describe how they meet the 6 family functions and tasks described in Chapter 16.

Family Health: Assessment and Practice

Learning Objectives

- Describe the effect of family health on individual health and community health.
- Describe individual and group characteristics of a healthy family.
- Describe three conceptual frameworks that can be used to asses a family.
- Describe the 12 major assessment categories for families.
- List the five basic principles the community health nurse should follow when assessing family health.

Key Terms

- Developmental framework
- Eco-map
- Family health
- Family nursing
- Genogram

- Interactional framework
- Social support network map
- Strengthening
- Structural-functional framework

Chapter Summary

Community health nurses have a long history of focusing on the family as a unity of service. They were aware of the significant influence the family had on an individual's health and therefore on the larger community. The focus has continued and today the family remains an emphasis of community health nursing services. There is a gap however, between family nursing theory, development, and practice. This is fostered in part by a health care delivery system that fosters the health of individuals, often to the exclusion of the family.

Families do not exist in isolation from the rest of the world. Healthy families influence their communities in a positive way, and conversely, unhealthy families have a negative effect.

Strengths of a healthy family include such things as family pride, support, cohesion, adaptability, communication, religious orientation, and social support (Olson, McCubbin, and Associates, 1983). Six important characteristics of a healthy family are:

1. There is a facilitative process of interaction among family members.

2. They enhance individual development.

3. Their role relationships are structured effectively.

4. They actively attempt to cope with problems.

5. They have a healthy home environment and life- style.

6. They establish regular links with the broader community.

Each of these characteristics is discussed in detail in this chapter. In order to collect data related to the family's health practices and provide a comprehensive approach to assessing individual needs, the community health nurse needs to use five guidelines. These guidelines can clarify an understanding of family nursing and enhance practice with families.

1. Work with the family collectively.

2. Start where the family is.

3. Adapt nursing interventions to the family's stage of development.

4. Recognize the validity of variations in family structures.

5. Emphasize family strengths.

In order to assist the nurse in a systematic assessment of family health, three tools are used: a conceptual framework, a clearly defined set of assessment categories for data collection, and a method for measuring a family's level of functioning. Three conceptual frameworks used for studying families are discussed: the interactional framework, the structural-functional framework, and the developmental framework. As an initial framework for assessing family health, the six characteristics of a healthy family are used with the three other frameworks mentioned.

Useful data for assessing a family's health includes the following twelve categories: demographics, physical environment, psychological and spiritual environment, family structure and role, functions, values and beliefs, communication patterns, decision-making patterns, problem-solving patterns, coping patterns, family health behavior, and family social and cultural patterns.

In family assessment the community health nurse focuses on the family, not the member, using goal-directed questions, allowing adequate time for data collection, combining quantitative and qualitative data, and exercising professional judgement. Graphic assessment tools used by the community health nurse generate information about selected aspects of family structure and function. These tools include the ecomap, genogram and social network support map. A classic model for family nursing by Tapia (1972) includes five levels of family functioning and appropriate nursing roles. Two assessment tools are also discussed to assist the nurse with data collection.

Teaching Strategies

A. Classroom Strategies

1. Provide the students with the five case studies in this chapter (or other case studies the faculty member might choose) and have the students identify some healthy characteristics and unhealthy characteristics of these families. Describe how the health or illness of the families could influence the health of their communities.

2. Have a school nurse or another community health nurse discuss with the class how family relationships and family health practices influence a child's ability to perform academically and to interact effectively with peers.

B. Clinical Laboratory Strategies

1. Ask students to use the family assessment tools in the text to study a family or families as part of their community assessment.
2. Ask students to complete an ecomap and/or genogram of one of the families in their community assessment assignment.

Evaluation Strategies

A. Multiple Choice Questions

1. What is an ecomap?
   a. A diagram of family relationships over three or more generations
   b. A diagram of connections between the family and other systems
   c. A chart that depicts the ecological system of a family's neighborhood
   d. A map that provides directions to the neighborhood where data is to be gathered

2. In the Levels of Family Functioning Model by Tapia the family in childhood (Level II) is
   a. slightly above survival level with limited ability to trust.
   b. an average family with more than its share of problems.
   c. a well family functioning independently.
   d. very chaotic and barely surviving.

3. The nurse working with the Beck family (depicted in the text) is an example of how the nurse
   a. starts where the family is.
   b. adapts intervention according to the family's stage of development.
   c. recognizes the validity of family structure variations.
   d. works with the family collectively.

4. How does an interactional framework describe the family?
   a. As a social system relating to other social systems
   b. From a life-cycle perspective
   c. In terms of the characteristics of a healthy family
   d. By looking at the interacting personalities between family members

5. Which of the following is the best way to conduct an accurate family assessment?
   a. Making several visits and accumulating data from all family members
   b. Using quantitative data only to maintain and preserve objectivity
   c. Questioning one family member to avoid confusion and repeated information
   d. Use a questionnaire format, and complete the tool in the family's presence

B. True/False Questions

1. A genogram is a diagram of family relationships over three or more generations.
   a. True
   b. False

2. In the Tapia model, the Level V family receives the greatest amount of services from the community health nurse.
   a. True
   b. False

3. A healthy family can remain isolated from the broader community.
   a. True
   b. False

4. The developmental framework studies families from a life-cycle perspective.
   a. True
   b. False

5. To enhance care to clients, the community health nurse must start at where the family is.
   a. True
   b. False

C. Essay Questions

1. Using the data collection method in table 17-1, assess your own family including the twelve assessment categories.

2. Using two of the five case studies in this chapter, assess them for their level of health using the six characteristics for a healthy family on page 368.

D. Individual or Group Projects

1. Ask students to assess their own family through the use of a genogram and share it with the student group verbally. Each student should bring samples of family photos and identify ages and causes of death among deceased family members. Do any specific patterns emerge? Discuss observations.

2. Among a specified number of students or in one clinical laboratory group, assess each assigned client family according to the Tapia Model presented in this chapter. In what levels do most families function? What does this mean for the role of the nurse and types of services provided?

18

Promoting and Protecting the Health of Maternal, Prenatal, and Newborn Populations

Learning Objectives

- Identify the health goals established by the U.S. Department of Health and Human Services in 1990 for the maternal-infant population.
- Discuss the major risk factors for pregnant women and infants.
- Describe the important considerations in designing good health promotion programs to fit the needs of diverse maternal-infant populations.
- List several features of a typical health promotion program for maternal-infant populations.
- Identify several methods of delivering services to maternal-infant populations.
- Describe the different roles of a community health nurse in serving the maternal-infant population.

Key Terms

- Continuous quality improvement
- Drug dependent
- Drug exposed
- Fetal alcohol effects
- Fetal alcohol syndrome
- High-risk infants
- Low birth weight
- Passive smoking
- Self-help group
- Smokeless tobacco products
- Very low birth weight

Chapter Summary

Providing effective primary prevention services for pregnant women, new mothers, and infants presents many challenges for the community health nurse. Chapter 18 identifies influences on the health of these populations and their specific needs. The development of maternal and infant health programs, community resources, and the different roles of the community health nurse working to improve the maternal and infant health are the focus in this chapter.

Vital statistics of the past decade indicate that the United States has made strides in improving maternal and infant health. However, infant mortality rates are still significantly above the "Healthy People 2000" goals set by the U.S. Public Health Service in 1990 and remain higher than those of 21 other nations. Low-birthweight infants account for two-thirds of the infant deaths in this country.

Lifestyle factors, sociodemographic forces, and medical-gestational history contribute most to the health problems of pregnant women and infants. Community health nurses can have the greatest impact in the area of teaching women to avoid making unhealthy life-style choices. Alcohol use, cigarette smoking, exposure to STDs and the HIV virus, and maternal weight gain are issues in which community health nursing interventions can have a significant influence. Infants born to teenagers are at high risk for neonatal and postneonatal mortality. Almost 11,000 infants were born to teens under 15 years of age in 1990 and 350,000 to 15-19 year old teens (Statistical Abstracts of U.S., 1993). Maternal and infant health related programs will remain a focus of attention for our nation for decades to come. Each of these categories of factors are explored in this chapter.

Successful health care programs organized and delivered in a logical manner can result from coordinated community planning. Valuable time and resources are saved by appropriate distribution and use of services. Accessible services that are based on identified needs and developmental stage of the population are utilized the best. The federal government has been granting money to states for the promotion of maternal and child health. These grants supplement state funds to meet maternal and child health care needs at the local level. The implementation of programs is different in each state and community based on funding, staffing, and geographic distribution of clients and their needs. Services are delivered through clinics, home visits, self-help groups (Chapter 10), school-based programs (Chapter 19) and high risk clinics.

Qualified nursing personnel are required if such programs are to be effective. Three aspects are emphasized when working with the maternal and infant population: 1) special professional qualities, 2) competence in the role of educator, and 3) extensive use of the role of client advocate and liaison. A working knowledge of community resources for assistance and referral is essential, such as the department of social services, Supplemental Food

Program for Women, Infants, and Children (WIC), family planning services, and childbirth education classes.

A carefully designed, systematic plan for evaluation of maternal-infant health programs should be developed. The answers to the following questions will assist in the evaluation process:

- Did the program meet the identified needs of the population?

- Did it meet identified goals and objectives?

- Was the program cost-effective?

- What was the program's long-term impact of the health of this population?

Evaluation data can be obtained from vital statistics, quality management systems, and audits of client records.

As we enter the twenty-first century there will be an increased demand for the community health nurse to obtain grant funding to finance programs and to develop new programs for a more complex client population.

Teaching Strategies

A. Classroom Strategies

1. Supply the class with the vital statistics for your city, county and/or state and have the students compare and contrast these statistics with the national statistics provided on page 394 of this chapter. Discuss possible reasons for either a higher or lower infant mortality in your city, county and/or state.

2. Hold a brainstorming session (Chapter 13) to generate a list of factors contributing to infant mortality and low-birthweight infants in your community. From this list, have the class develop a community program to address these factors.

B. Clinical Laboratory Strategies

1. Have the students prepare a teaching plan on a topic related to antepartum or postpartum nursing care. The plan should include objectives, topic content, teacher-learner activities including audio-visual materials and/or handouts, method of teaching, and method for evaluation. Provide the students with an

opportunity to present their class to a group of pregnant or postpartum women and their families. Refer to Chapter 14 for teaching strategies, if this content has not been covered previously.

2. Have students locate a self-help group working with a maternal and infant population and attend a meeting. The students should return to the clinical laboratory group and be prepared to present to their peers the goals and accomplishments of the group. Do this early in the clinical course so that the students will have information about support groups to share with clients during the span of the course.

Evaluation Strategies

A. Multiple Choice Questions

1. In the United States the infant mortality rate for 1990
    a. is 14.1 per 1000 live births.
    b. is lower than those of France, Italy and Japan.
    c. continued to rise for African-American infants.
    d. is higher than those of 21 other countries.

2. The most productive role for the community health nurse working with the maternal and infant population is that of
    a. counselor.
    b. advocate.
    c. educator.
    d. liaison.

3. Ineffective or failed community health care projects are often the result of
    a. designing a plan to meet specific identified needs.
    b. incomplete assessment and lack of involvement of targeted populations.
    c. failure to use a predetermined, generalized plan for all those served.
    d. identifying the developmental stage of the population being served.

4. Alcohol consumption during pregnancy has been MOST associated with infant
    a. intellectual impairment.
    b. low birth-weight.
    c. respiratory distress.
    d. childhood cancers.

5. Smoking during pregnancy has been MOST associated with infant
   a. genetic malformations.
   b. low birth-weight.
   c. developmental delays.
   d. feeding problems.

B. True/False Questions

1. In a self-help group, individuals regain their sense of identity and control.
   a. True
   b. False

2. FAE is three times more common than FAS.
   a. True
   b. False

3. The HIV virus does not transmit to infants through breast milk.
   a. True
   b. False

4. Infants born to drug exposed or drug dependent women is a minor problem in the United States.
   a. True
   b. False

5. Federal monies help to support state maternal and child health programs.
   a. True
   b. False

C. Essay Questions

1. Reflect on the pregnant women you have provided care to in the nursing program thus far. What high risk behaviors (discussed in this chapter) did you observe in your clients? Did you discuss the behaviors with the clients? Did they change their high risk behavior? What would you do differently now that you are taking community health nursing?

2. Reflect on the pregnancy of a person you know personally. What behaviors did she display that may be considered high risk? Did you discuss the behaviors with

her? Did any of her behaviors change? How different are people you know personally than pregnant clients you have cared for?

D. Individual or Group Projects

1. Arrange for a group of students to visit the local regional, or county health department or other community agencies providing maternal- infant services and to meet with the director of those services. Questions that the students could ask the director might include the following:

   - How many clients are served?

   - What are the demographic and socioeconomic statistics of the clients?

   - How do the clients qualify for prenatal are?

   - What are the primary health concerns of women attending the clinic?

   - What are the infant outcomes for women seen for prenatal care?

   Give a report to the entire class on the findings.

2. Arrange opportunities for students to teach a class or a series of classes on maternal and infant care (see Chapter 14 on teaching strategies). There are many community sites where maternal and infant populations gather including; clinics, WIC centers, childbirth education classes, nurse-midwife, nurse practitioner or physician offices.

Promoting and Protecting the Health of Toddler, Preschool, School-Age, and Adolescent Populations

19

Learning Objectives

- Identify major health problems, and concerns for toddler, pre-school, school-age, and adolescent populations in the Untied States.
- Explain the programs that promote health and prevent illness of toddler, pre-school, school-age, and adoloescent populations.
- State the recommended immunization schedule for children from birth through the teen years and give the rationale of the timing of each immunization.
- Describe the three functions of school nursing practice (health services, health education, and improvement of the school environment).
- Give examples of methods the community health nurse might use in working with toddlers, pre-school, school-age, and adolescents to help promote their health.

Key Terms

- Anorexia nervosa
- Attention Deficit Disorder (without hyperactivity) (ADD)
- Attention Deficit Hyperactivity Disorder (ADHD)
- Bulimia
- Child abuse
- High risk families
- School nurse
- School nurse practitioner

Chapter Summary

Knowledge and skills related to children's health problems are important components of community health nursing. Chapter 19 begins with a discussion of the drop in childhood mortality rates in this country and the reasons for the change. While infectious diseases once caused the majority of childhood deaths, accidents are now the leading cause of death for children age 1-14. An increasing cause of deaths for children and teens is violence within the community and death by handguns, drug overdose, and AIDS. A disturbing constant is a high morbidity rate among children. There is an increased awareness of learning disorders and emotional behavioral problems related to maternal drug use, dysfunctional families, lead poisoning, and violence.

Health concerns for the various age groups of children are discussed, along with known causes of children's diseases and accidents leading to trauma. The toddler (the one and two year old child) and pre-school population (the three and four year old child) have low mortality but high morbidity. Frequent acute illnesses account for a large number of days of restricted activity and disability. This age group is especially prone to falls, burns, and poisonings. Nutritional, dental health, and mental health needs are great as they rapidly grow toward school age.

Mortality is also low in the school age population (the five to fourteen year old child). Motor vehicle accidents lead the causes of death list for this age group. Morbidity from respiratory illnesses, parasitic diseases, injuries, and digestive conditions remains high. Communicable disease incidences from preventable diseases has dropped considerably because of widespread immunization efforts. There are many children however, who are unimmunized or underimmunized. Vigorous immunization campaigns have been tentatively effective. Behavioral and learning problems among school aged children are becoming recognized more frequently by families, school officials and health care providers. ADHD and ADD descriptions are included in Table 19-1, p. 416. Nutrition and dental health problems continue to affect this age group in large numbers, especially among specific cultural groups.

The adolescent population has mortality rates 2.5 times higher than younger children. The death rate has been gradually increasing since 1960 (U.S. Dept. of Commerce, 1993). Adolescent health problems are varied and complex. Major issues include emotional problems and suicide, violence, substance abuse, pregnancy, STDs and HIV/AIDS and poor nutrition and eating habits.

Services for children are grouped in categories of preventative health, health protection, and health promotion. Preventative health programs include quality day care, accessible immunization programs, and education and social services. Health protection programs include safety and injury prevention, child protection services (at three levels of prevention), and oral hygiene and dental care. Health promotion programs include day care and pre-school programs, nutrition and exercise programs, education to prevent substance abuse, and counseling and crisis intervention.

School health nursing practice is described in detail and seeks to improve the health of children through health education, provision of health services, and promotion of a healthful environment in the school system. The school nurse works as a liaison with the interdisciplinary school health team. The complex role of school nurse is best accomplished through special training and the development of advanced skills. The uniqueness of the school nurse role is highlighted through the case study on Ellen Ramsey.

Teaching Strategies

A. Classroom Strategies

1. Obtain vital statistics on children ages 1-18 for your community and state. Compare the mortality and morbidity rates against the goals in "Healthy People 2000." Determine how close your local community and state comes to meeting the national health objectives.

2. Assess students for their willingness to share personal information about themselves, siblings and their own children. If they are receptive, discuss the group's personal experiences with childhood mortality and morbidity. Does the distribution compare with those issues highlighted in Chapter 19? Discuss differences and contemplate why there are differences.

B. Clinical Laboratory Strategies

1. Have the students spend an observational/participatory day with local school nurses at the elementary and high school levels. Compare and contrast school nursing roles during a clinical laboratory conference.

2. Have students plan and present a health promotion program for preschool children in a day-care setting or Head Start program.

Evaluation Strategies

A. Multiple Choice Questions

1. The major cause of death in children in the United States is
   a. pneumonia.
   b. infectious diseases.
   c. poverty.
   d. accidents.

2. What is the primary cause of nutritional problems among school-age children?
   a. Living in the culture of poverty
   b. Cultural food preferences
   c. Experiencing growth spurts
   d. Overeating and inappropriate food choices

3. The community health nurse's role in providing health services for children involves organizing programs for prevention of illness and injury, promotion of good health practices, and protection of health. Which of the following interventions would be classified as protection?
   a. Immunization programs
   b. Comprehensive preschool programs
   c. Case finding and reporting
   d. Nutrition and weight-reduction programs

4. Which of the following is the leading health problem among adolescents?
   a. Violent death and injury
   b. Suicide
   c. Infectious diseases
   d. Sexually transmitted diseases

5. Signs and symptoms of a child with ADD include
   a. fidgeting and squirming when sitting.
   b. talking excessively.
   c. difficulty playing quietly.
   d. daydreaming and lack of follow through.

B. True/False Questions

1. School-age children experience more acute disorders than other populations.
   a. True
   b. False

2. Approximately 5% of school-age children have learning disabilities and behavior problems.
   a. True
   b. False

3. Firearm violence is the leading cause of death for 15-19 year old black males.
   a. True
   b. False

4. Suicide rates for adolescents doubled during the 20 years between 1970-1990.
   a. True
   b. False

5. The World Health Organization reports that in many countries 25% of new HIV infections are among 15-24 year olds.
   a. True
   b. False

C. Essay Questions

1. In 200 words or less complete the following thought and describe what you would do to fulfill the role. "If I were a school nurse I would....."

2. Identify the levels of prevention for teenage suicide.

D. Individual or Group Projects

1. Have a small group of students plan a health and safety fair at a local school. The students would need to meet with school officials, complete a needs assessment, contact appropriate agencies to participate in the fair and plan the day and location of the event. This same activity can be planned by 3-4 groups at schools with different age children (pre-school, elementary, middle-school, and high school).

2. Arrange for students interested in school nursing to spend some of their clinical laboratory hours with a school nurse and have sufficient involvement to participate in all aspects of the school nursing role. Community health clinical laboratory objectives can be met in this setting and many school nurses will welcome the opportunity to share their expertise.

20 Promoting and Protecting the Health of Adults and the Working Population

Learning Objectives

- Describe major events in the historical development of occupational health nursing.
- Discuss significant legislation affecting occupational health and safety.
- Identify potential physical, chemical, biological, ergonomic, and psychosocial stressors in a variety of work environments.
- Explain several types of occupational health programs related to health protection, health prevention, and health promotion.
- Describe the role of occupational health team members in a multi-disciplinary approach to worker health and safety.
- Describe how experts believe the practice of occupational health nursing will change to meet future needs within a changing health care delivery system.

Key Terms

- Disabled person
- Ergonomics
- Job burnout
- Job stress
- Line position
- Migrant worker
- Nonoccupational injuries and illness
- Occupational health
- Staff position
- Universal precautions
- Work stressors
- Workers

Chapter Summary

During the last quarter of the 20th century, the American labor force changed in composition. Once made up primarily of male blue-collar workers, it has shifted to include a majority of white-collar workers. Forty-six percent of the country's workers are now female (U.S. Bureau of Census, 1993). Chapter 20 discusses five environmental factors common to every work setting that influence the health of workers. The factors are physical, chemical, biological, ergonomic, and psychosocial.

Physical aspects of the work environment include the work space, temperature, lighting, noise, vibration, color, radiation, pressure, and soundness of the building and equipment. Depending on the type of work and place of work, one or many of these factors may place the worker at risk.

Chemicals in the workplace can affect employees working as dry cleaners, painters, photographers, auto manufacturers, farmers, pharmaceutical manufacturers, and hospital employees. Chemicals are present in many forms: gases, solvents, mists, vapors, dusts, and solids. They can enter the human body through the lungs, gastrointestinal tract, and/or skin. Diseases related to exposure to chemicals may take years to develop and the worker may not be aware of the insidious onset of some chemically induced diseases. Some workers are exposed to bacteria viruses, rickettsiae, molds, fungi and various parasites and toxic plants. Workers especially at risk are farmers, slaughterhouse workers, and various outdoor workers.

Ergonomic factors are the concerns for the design of the workplace. At times the actual worksetting, tools the worker must use, and position they must get into to complete the job contribute to ergonomic problems in the work setting.

Psychological stresssors occur in some settings. Some work tasks may be in conflict with a worker's values and/or ethics. The job may cause the employee to be fatigued, angry, bored, tense, depressed or agitated. No one goes to work expecting to come home ill or injured because of job requirements, but this happens to thousands of Americans each day.

Historically workers had deplorable conditions at work and were exploited. As the United States became increasingly more industrialized, significant legislation was enacted. The Workmen's Compensation Act of 1911, the Social Security Act of 1935, the Federal Coal Mine Health and Safety Act of 1967, the Occupational Safety and Health Act of 1970, the Privacy Act of 1974, the Toxic Substances Control Act of 1976, the Hazard Communication Act of 1986, the American with Disabilities Act of 1990, and the OSHA Bloodborne Pathogen Standard of 1992 are some of the most significant pieces of legislation protecting workers in the United States.

Lung disease, injuries, and occupational cancers are the leading work-associated health disorders. Apart from health problems related to the work environment, heart disease, cancer, and stroke are the three leading causes of death among the adult population. Table 20-2, p. 447, shows the statistics. Many of the causes of death are acquired in the work setting by exposure to substances previously mentioned. The leading health problems of American adults aged 25 to 64 are accidents, cancer, heart disease, suicide, and HIV virus (U.S. Statistical Abstracts, 1994). Chronic diseases pose the most significant threat to the health of American adults.

Programs designed to address occupational safety and health focus on prevention, protection, and health promotion. Such programs are administered by community health nurses working in occupational settings in collaboration with other occupational health and safety professionals. The special skills and demands of the occupational health nurse focus on the changing health care delivery system. A case study is presented demonstrating the comprehensiveness of the occupational health nursing role as carried out by Victor Ramos.

Teaching Strategies

A. Classroom Strategies

1. Have students share known occupational illness/injuries among their own family members. Do they relate more to health problems acquired in workers 20, 30, or 40 years ago than those younger family members working now? What makes the difference in the numbers and types of illnesses or injuries?

2. Invite an occupational health nurse to speak to the class about his/her role.

B. Clinical Laboratory Strategies

1. Suggest that students spend an observational day with an occupational health nurse to observe workers' health programs and the nurse's role in those programs.

2. Tour a large manufacturing plant with an occupational health nurse and have the clinical laboratory students identify potential and actual safety hazards, protective devises used, and health and safety programs for the employees. Discuss the group's observations during a clinical laboratory conference.

Evaluation Strategies

A. Multiple Choice Questions

1. Every workplace has physical, chemical, biological, ergonomical, and psychosocial factors that affect workers' health. Examples of ergonomical factors related to the worksite are such things as:
   a. temperature, light, noise, or vibration.
   b. solvents, mists, vapors, or dusts.
   c. human interaction with workplace design, tools, tasks, and equipment.
   d. fatigue, anger, boredom versus enthusiasm, energy, and challenge.

2. The category of employees most exposed to bacteria, fungi, viruses, and molds include
   a. auto manufacturers.
   b. painters.
   c. photographers.
   d. farmers.

3. Today's workers are protected by such significant legislation as the Workman's Compensation Act of 1911 and the Occupational Safety and Health Act of 1970. Which of the following is one aspect of the latter (OSHA)?
   a. Provides black lung benefits to aged and disabled coal miners
   b. Protects workers against injury and illness resulting from hazardous working conditions
   c. Provides injured workers with medical and rehabilitative care
   d. Protects the privacy of workers from federal agencies collecting data on individuals

4. Work-related injuries are known to affect more than 17 million workers in the United States each year, and contributes to an estimated 99,000 work-related deaths annually. Some other health-related problems present a concern to health care workers because
   a. for many illnesses there is a lag time between exposure, onset, and clinical evidence.
   b. industries are reluctant to report complaints of worker injuries.
   c. research methods are not developed enough to enable occupational health researchers to make predictions.
   d. workers hesitate to report complaints because of fear of losing their jobs.

5. The Americans with Disabilities Act of 1990 was passed to
   a. ensure that substances do not present an unreasonable health risk to workers.
   b. limit the type and amount of information released to the government about workers.
   c. prevent discrimination against qualified workers with disabilities.
   d. require employers to carry employee insurance.

B. True/False Questions

1. More workers are injured or killed at work today than 10 years ago.
   a. True
   b. False

2. A responsibility of NIOSH includes monitoring and enforcing regulations and standards.
   a. True
   b. False

3. A responsibility of OSHA includes requiring employers to keep accurate employee illness and injury records.
   a. True
   b. False

4. The Privacy Act of 1974 provides for separate and adequate toileting facilities for men and women.
   a. True
   b. False

5. The Social Security Act of 1935 provides financial resources to the "aged, blind, and disabled".
   a. True
   b. False

C. Essay Questions

1. Select one of the five environmental factors that affects you in your work. List the aspects of that factor that could affect your health and identify what you can do about them to change the situation.

2. Occupational health nurses are usually not employed by small companies, however, if you had a company with 50 employees and could "contract" for the services of an OHN 8 hours a week, what would you have the nurse focus on in the time allotted? Your company produces gourmet ice cream and operates 16 hours a day, 6 days a week.

D. Individual or Group Projects

1. Have a group of students complete an assessment on a small local company (with the company's cooperation) as an external review service. Determine the positive and negative aspects of the company's health and safety program. Share the results with the company OHN or safety director and classmates and make suggestions for safety improvements if necessary.

2. If students are presently employed in a health care setting suggest they assess their hospital unit, agency, or service for adequacy of health and safety standards. If hazards exist, the student should share the information with a supervisor. The students should write a report including the areas strengths and weaknesses.

Promoting and Protecting the Health of the Older Adult Population

Learning Objectives

- Describe the health status of older adults in the United States today.
- List some of the major misconceptions held about the older adult population.
- Describe the major health needs of the older population.
- Discuss four primary criteria for effective programs for older adults.
- Describe various living arrangements and care options for older adults.
- Describe the future role of the community health nurse when working with older adults.

Key Terms

- Ageism
- Alzheimer's Disease
- Assisted living
- Board and care homes
- Capable elderly
- Case management
- Confidant
- Continuing care centers
- Custodial care
- Frail elderly
- Geriatrics
- Gerontics
- Gerontology
- Group home
- Hearty elderly
- Hospice care
- Intermediate care
- Long-term care
- Personal care homes
- Respite care
- Senility
- Skilled-nursing facility

Chapter Summary

People aged 65 and older make up the fastest growing segment of the American population and the most rapid increase is expected in the first third of the 21st century. This group poses a special challenge for the community health nurse and Chapter 21 focuses on population-based nursing for older adults.

First this chapter examines characteristics of the aging population and looks at some misconceptions about elders. Next their health needs are explored. Finally, health services and nursing interventions are discussed in light of cost containment and comprehensive care.

The concepts of hearty elderly, capable elderly, and frail elderly are explored. Only about 5% of people over 65 are institutionalized and the others live independently needing assistance in meeting activities of daily living as they age. By the time adults are over 85 years old, 50% need regular assistance to maintain independence. Older adults are one of the most stereotyped groups and many misconceptions about them exist. Several misconceptions are explored in this chapter on pages 465-467.

Health needs of the older adult are often complicated by multiple chronic and disabling conditions and their needs should be identified and met. Nutritional and exercise needs, psychosocial needs (which include coping with multiple losses, economic security needs and need for independence), needs of those with chronic health conditions of Alzheimers' disease, COPD, and CVAs are common needs of elders. Each can be complicated by multiple drug interactions and side effects. A final need of older adults is to plan for death.

The community health perspective includes the three disciplines of geriatrics, gerontology, and gerontics (each is described), and case management and needs assessment. The community health perspective of care must concern itself with the group of elderly as a whole, such as those in adult day care centers, those in a retirement community, or those using the services of meals on wheels.

Health programs for the elderly need to encompass the full range of needed services. This includes being financially and physically accessible and encouraging self-care and independence. Effective services for older adults meet four criteria. They are comprehensive, coordinated, accessible, and provide quality services. Services for older adults include living arrangements and care options such as facilities offering nursing care: skilled, intermediate skilled, and assisted care. There is also personal care, board and care, and group homes. Each offers a different set of living arrangements and services based on the needs of the older adult. The new and growing phenomenon of continuing care centers is explored and an example of one is shared in Display 21-4. Additional services to assist seniors remain at home as long as possible are discussed and include home care, day care, respite, and hospice services.

This chapter ends with a discussion of the future roles community health nurses will encounter as our society ages. Larger numbers of older adults need extensive multi-faceted services and community health nurses will need to be prepared to meet the goals "Healthy People 2000" established for the elderly.

Teaching Strategies

A. Classroom Strategies

1. Have students describe their perceptions of elderly persons. They can do this by writing poems or short essays. Simply give them the title of "older people" as an assignment. Have the poems copied and distributed to each student (with permission of the students), and discuss the feelings and perceptions described in the poems.

2. Invite elderly members of the community to speak to the class. Discuss the following topics:
   a. life-style changes caused by aging
   b. health needs
   c. social support systems
   d. hobbies and recreational activities
   e. transportation problems, if any
   f. perceptions about how others feel about aging and how they feel about their own aging
   (add additional topics relevant to your community)

B. Clinical Laboratory Strategies

1. Have students carry out the following activities:
   a. Complete a community assessment to gather data on the elderly population, and prioritize the identified needs.
   b. Speak to a member of the local police force regarding safety problems of seniors.
   c. Speak to a representative of the department of Health and Human Services regarding elder abuse, economic security, and alternatives to institutional care.

2. Have students use data obtained from the vital statistics of a predetermined census tract and other community sources to determine the following information:
   a. The number of elderly people in the community
   b. Where the elderly live (location, type of housing)
   c. The needs of the following age groups in areas such as health, recreation, transportation, etc. (65-74, 75-84, 85 and older)

Evaluation Strategies

A. Multiple Choice Questions

1. One important task that nurses should perform in working with an elderly population in the community is
    a. placing the elderly in nursing homes so they can be provided with the best care available.
    b. developing case management programs to channel clients to appropriate services.
    c. raising funds to support the needs of the elderly in the community.
    d. emphasizing tertiary prevention at this stage in the lives of the elderly.

2. Chronic diseases are common among older adults. Select the statement that most accurately reflects older adults and chronic diseases.
    a. Postural hypotension can cause falls in elders.
    b. Twenty percent of older adults can be considered hypertensive.
    c. Postural hypertension is a safety problem for elders.
    d. Older white men have the highest rates of hypertension.

3. The nursing care and services provided to seniors is a description of the focus of
    a. geriatrics.
    b. gerontology.
    c. gerontics.
    d. case management.

4. Continuing care centers
    a. provide housing and care as needed to older adults.
    b. only accept clients needing skilled nursing services.
    c. are similar to board and care homes.
    d. are respite centers for family members of older adults.

5. Specific goals of "Healthy People 2000" for older adults include
    a. promoting longevity.
    b. assisting elders in finding leisure-time activities.
    c. decreasing urinary incontinence.
    d. reducing deaths from suicides.

B. True/False Questions

1. Many elderly people are confused and may be described in medical diagnostic terminology as senile.
   a. True
   b. False

2. Older people have a tendency to disengage from productive life after retirement.
   a. True
   b. False

3. The older adult's exercise needs decrease with age, and being sedentary is a healthier choice.
   a. True
   b. False

4. Mortality after bereavement is high for older adults.
   a. True
   b. False

5. Independence helps to meet the need for self-respect and dignity.
   a. True
   b. False

C. Essay Questions

1. Using the phrase, "When I am 85 years old, I will......". Complete your thoughts in as much detail as possible.

2. Describe briefly an older adult you know. Develop a health promotion plan for them based on strategies for successful aging proposed by Bortz(1991).

D. Individual or Group Projects

1. Interview a group of seniors at a senior center as part of a needs assessment for the agency. What wants and needs do the participants identify? Which ones can a community health nurse help to meet?

2. Using the information gathered in activity #1, plan several programs to meet the needs and wants of the attendees at the senior center.

22 Promoting and Protecting the Health of the Home Care Population

Learning Objectives

- Define home health care.
- Describe the evolution of home care services to the present.
- Describe the range of services provided to clients by home health agencies.
- Compare and contrast community health nursing and home health nursing.
- Explain the future of the nurses' role in the home care movement including concepts of quality improvement/assurance, case management, and managed care.

Key Terms

- Home health care
- Homebound
- Homemakers
- Hospital-based home health agency
- Official home health agency
- Proprietary home health agency
- Voluntary home health agency

Chapter Summary

In this chapter home health care is broadly defined as "all services and products provided to clients in their homes to maintain, restore, or promote their physical, mental, and emotional health." Home health care assists clients attaining their highest possible levels of independence by helping them maintain their independence at home, which is preferred, and avoiding or postponing institutionalization. The major subpopulations for home health care are older adults living at home, long-term care clients who are not institutionalized, discharged acute care clients, and people who are interested in wellness and self-care.

Because home health care has a broad spectrum of clients, the services needed by clients in their homes vary. Home health care is becoming more complex as clients are discharged from hospitals sooner, are more acutely ill, or may have undergone surgery in an outpatient setting and need follow-up from specialized health care providers. Care at home may include nursing, medical and dental care, pharmaceutical services, social services counseling, physical therapy, speech therapy, occupational therapy, laboratory testing, nutrition education, homemaker or home health aide services, provision of equipment and supplies, chore services, health screening, and information on illness prevention. Several organizations are particularly concerned about providing quality home care. They include the National League for Nursing, the National Association of Home Health Agencies, the American Hospital Association, and others.

The history of home health care in the United States dates back to the 1800s, when such care was organized by laypersons. In 1877, the Women's Branch of the New York City Mission was the first group to employ a graduate nurse to deliver home care. In 1893, Lillian Wald established the visiting Nurse Service of New York City. Between that time and the beginning of World War II, nurses and physicians worked together to provide health care to people in their homes. Physician shortages during World War II meant that the limited number of available physicians saw clients mainly in hospitals and doctors' offices, and physicians moved out of the arena of home health care. For about two decades most of the home health care provided in the United States was administered by visiting nurse associations or outreach services offered through some hospitals. The primary clients were elderly people with chronic illnesses who required a combination of nursing care and personal services. Payment was made by welfare or by clients themselves on a sliding fee scale subsidized by charity or the agency providing the service.

The advent of Medicare and Medicaid legislation in 1965 changed the system tremendously in regard to client eligibility and payment source. The federal government began to appoint physicians to direct the traditionally nonmedical home services, and home care changed to a medical-based model of practice. To be eligible for Medicare coverage, a home care client had to be referred by a physician who certified that they were in need of skilled care and are essentially homebound. Medicare and Medicaid did not provide reimbursement for preventive, health-promoting, or support services. Reimbursement is still very limited in these areas.

Millions of people in America today need some type of home health service. Forces promoting the growth of home health care include cost containment pressures by the government, third-party payers, and employers; an expanding elderly population; lack of family-member caregivers because more women work outside the home and family members live distant from one another; consumer demands for greater satisfaction and quality of life; and new technology that makes it possible to maintain greater numbers of ill and disabled people outside the hospital setting. To meet the needs of home health clients, for-profit and voluntary agencies now offer a broad range of services and supplies. In some cases, supply companies are attempting joint ventures with hospital-based home health services. This is a change from the past, when home health services were usually provided by nonprofit agencies.

The mix of home health care clients is changing. Half of all home care recipients are older than 65 and are visited in their homes (houses, apartments, continuing care centers, and retirement communities). Two-thirds are women. Disabled infants and children make up a growing number of home health clients. Clients with AIDS are being treated with life prolonging medications over extended periods of time. Because the home care population is dramatically changing, their needs are also changing and they fall into five categories: chronic illness and disability care, social support and interaction, alternative housing options, personal services and day care, and financial support or reimbursement. Home health care services available today are divided into three categories: 1) professional services, 2) support services, and 3) supplies and equipment. Not all services are paid for by third party reimbursement and the intensive home care needs of some clients require increased out of pocket payments.

Designing relevant, cost effective, and quality home care services depends on appropriately focused needs assessments and innovative thought. Several examples of programs that demonstrate creativity and cost savings are shared in this chapter. Special services of hospice care, long-term assistive services, and mental health care are being provided by many home health agencies to remain competitive. Current trends in home health care include: more hospitals expanding into home health care as well as new and varied free- standing agencies, acute care and intensive at-home care, new client groups with AIDS, chronic illnesses managed at home such as clients with cancer, ventilator dependent, and those needing central-line medications and parenteral nutrition.

Community health nurses can provide case management (where care is examined by insurance companies for the most efficient yet highest quality care) to home health clients, design newer and more effective methods of delivering home health care, and be in the forefront of change in this expanding field.

Teaching Strategies

A. Classroom Strategies

1. Ask the director of a home health agency to speak to the class about the services provided by his or her agency.

2. Conduct a seminar that compares the philosophy of a for-profit home health agency with that of a public health department in the community. Compare and contrast the roles and functions each serves in the community.

B. Clinical Laboratory Strategies

1. Have students visit a private retirement village and compare the health care needs and services found in that situation to those of an elderly population living in low-income housing.

2. Ask students to assess the community for service providers who can implement home health care. They should find out what type of payment plan is required and what gaps in service exist.

Evaluation Strategies

A. Multiple Choice Questions

1. The Visiting Nurse Service of New York City was founded by Lillian Wald in 1893 as
   a. a Red Cross unit whose nurses visited the sick, well babies, and school children.
   b. a hospital-based home care program at Montefiore hospital in New York.
   c. the first organized home nursing service in the United States.
   d. a home nursing service for Metropolitan Life Insurance Company's New York policy holders.

2. Medicare and Medicaid legislation enacted in 1965 drastically changed the home health care delivery system. What is the major change resulting from this legislation?

    a. Chronically ill elderly people now pay for services by sliding scale fees or charitable funds

    b. Physicians have not directed the home health care services since 1965

    c. The payment source changed, as did standards for determining client eligibility

    d. Home care is based on a nursing model rather than the medical model

3. A "certainty" about our health care delivery system is that

    a. change is inevitable.

    b. the amount of technical care will taper off.

    c. our present model of care will continue.

    d. home care demands will decrease in the future.

4. One part of a system to improve quality care is to

    a. continue nursing practice as usual if there are no major complaints.

    b. have clients complete a questionnaire after discharge from services.

    c. change agency philosophy to match available resources.

    d. keep client data that is gathered to a minimum to promote confidentiality.

5. How do home health nursing service clients differ from community health clients?

    a. Community health service clients are older than the home health care client population

    b. Home health care client needs are greater than community health client needs

    c. Home health care is provided to larger groups than in the community health setting

    d. Home health clients have skilled needs as determined by Medicare or Medicaid guidelines

B. True/False Questions

1. Home care is growing rapidly as a result of a cost containment focus in the heath care system.

    a. True

    b. False

2. The largest segment of the home care population is the maternal/infant population.
   a. True
   b. False

3. Home care services had its origins in the 1800s.
   a. True
   b. False

4. AIDS clients receive life prolonging treatments at home through home care services.
   a. True
   b. False

5. Medicare covers all home care needs of older adults.
   a. True
   b. False

C. Essay Questions

1. In your own words explain the difference between home health care service clients and community health nursing service clients.

2. How do you envision health care in the year 2020 and what will the home health care client profile look like?

D. Individual or Group Projects

1. Ask the director of a home health agency to allow you to participate in a chart audit on some clients. How does it differ from chart audits on hospitalized clients? Share this experience with classmates if all students were not involved. If all students were involved, compare and contrast agency protocol.

2. If a group of students made home visits to home health care clients have them share information about clients visited with common diagnoses (e.g., diabetes, CHF, CVA, etc.). Discuss how the agencies are managing client care. What supports do the clients have? How different is the support each client receives from families and friends? What makes the difference in their ability to manage well? How can the home care nurse make a difference in clients' response to illness and follow-up care?

Promoting Community Health Through Control of Communicable Diseases

Learning Objectives

- Explain the significance and use of surveillance methods in communicable disease control.
- List sources of food and water-borne disease.
- Describe control strategies for vector-borne diseases.
- Discuss specific ways to prevent sexually transmitted diseases, including HIV/AIDS.
- Differentiate between HIV infection and AIDS.
- Explain the significance of immunization as a communicable disease control measure.
- Describe the nurse's role in contact investigation.
- Discuss ethical issues affecting communicable disease and infection control.

Key Terms

- Acquired immunodeficiency syndrome (AIDS)
- Active immunity
- Communicable disease
- Direct transmission
- Endemic
- Epidemic
- Herd Immunity
- Human immunodeficiency virus (HIV)
- Immunization
- Incubation period
- Indirect transmission
- Infection
- Isolation
- Pandemic
- Passive immunity

- Quarantine
- Reservoir
- Screening

- Surveillance Vaccine
- Vaccine
- Vector

Chapter Summary

In Chapter 23 there is an expanded view of major communicable diseases affecting aggregates in the United States. For centuries communicable diseases have posed a major threat to the public's health and continues to challenge health care providers today. Some diseases are new in the last quarter of this century (HIV/AIDS), some are resurging and causing new problems (STDs and tuberculosis), and others are occurring in smaller numbers or disappearing due to our ability to vaccinate new generations against old and familiar diseases (measles and chickenpox). This chapter looks specifically at the communicable diseases needing to be controlled and hopefully eliminated.

Communicable diseases are transmitted directly from person to person or indirectly through a vector. They can have endemic, epidemic, or pandemic status as they exist and spread among populations. Assessing the communicable disease status of communities is accomplished through surveillance methods. It involves three steps: 1) systematic collection of data on specific diseases, 2) analysis and interpretation of data, and 3) dissemination of compiled and processed data for the purpose of program interventions. Collecting accurate data can be challenging. If the infected person does not require or can't afford medical intervention or if the health care worker does not follow through on their obligation to report certain illnesses, diseases can go vastly underreported.

Food and water-borne diseases, vector-borne diseases, and common infectious diseases where transmission is not directly person to person, are discussed. An agent in food or water, or insects, can cause illnesses that can be mild and more of a nuisance, or that can be life threatening. Control measures are covered for each category of disease transmission.

The STDs: syphilis, gonorrhea, chlamydia, and genital herpes and warts, are discussed as the most common sexually transmitted diseases we face today. The incidence, control efforts, and descriptions of the disease process for each of these STDs is covered. Prevention of STDs among high risk groups, especially teens, needs to be approached using creative programs. Clinic services must be more abundant and accessible. Statistics on the sexual practices of teens indicate that STDs and associated control measures will be needed for many more decades. The community health nurse has a major role in the control of STDs.

Each of the following diseases are covered: HIV/AIDS, STDs, and tuberculosis. Included for each disease is an overview, the at-risk populations, incidence and prevalence, and most effective control, diagnostic, and treatment or caregiving measures.

Immunization as a primary prevention method has a long and productive history in the United States. Even though immunizations are accessible through private and public settings that are low cost or free, children remain underimmunized. The national goal of 90 percent immunization compliance by age two is still far from being a reality especially in some communities. An immunization schedule is in Table 23-6. Barriers to adequate immunization coverage include: religious, financial, social, cultural, and provider limitations. Race, culture, and specific population characteristics need to be considered when planning immunization programs. Table 23-8 outlines the steps for administering immunization clinics. Adult immunization programs should not be overlooked. Many vaccines are needed by adults at specific times and/or regularly such as: hepatitis B, adult DT, and flu, pneumonia, and tetanus vaccines.

Community education through the use of mass media is a cost effective way to reach multitudes in the community and to promote primary prevention. Creative educational strategies are needed to get the health message to the targeted high risk groups.

Screening for disease or secondary prevention is the next line of defense against communicable diseases. Screening tests must be reliable and valid, and have predictive value and yield. The tests must also meet nine epidemiologic criteria for detection of health problems. Contact investigation is a major component to the control of some diseases and becomes challenging if it involves a highly mobile and transient population. Tertiary prevention measures include isolation and quarantine. Safe handling of contaminated infectious wastes are of major importance in the control of communicable diseases. EPA requirements for medical waste disposal are for segregating waste into three categories: 1) sharps, 2) toxic and hazardous, regulated, or infectious fluids, and 3) other materials.

Communicable diseases often occur among high risk groups and need to be considered separately. Pregnant women and infants, day care children, the homeless population, the chronically mentally ill and disabled population, international travelers and refugees, the home care population and community health nurses are all susceptible to a variety of communicable diseases because of the nature of their circumstances and bear special consideration.

There are ethical issues in communicable disease and infection control that community health nurses must consider. Those discussed in this chapter include access to disease prevention and treatment services, enforced compliance with preventive measures; screening programs; privacy, confidentiality, and descrimination; and issues involving the health care worker who is infected with or is a carrier of an infectious disease.

Teaching Strategies

A. Classroom Strategies

1. Invite an epidemiologist/clinician from an STD clinic to discuss local trends in STD incidence and control. Perhaps the speaker has slides of classic and common STDs to enhance the presentation.

2. Invite the leader of an AIDS support group or a family and friends of AIDS clients' support group to talk to the class. Ask the speaker to focus on the role of the nurse that he/she feels is most important when working with AIDS clients.

B. Clinical Laboratory Strategies

1. Encourage students to spend clinical laboratory time in an STD clinic in a participatory (preferred) or observer role. Their main objective should be to explore the care provider's role, caregiving technique, and counseling style. The students should write a critique of this experience in a journal.

2. Allow students to participate in an immunization clinic. Provide an inservice on immunization administration (if needed or as review) and have students participate in well-baby immunization clinics, flu clinics for older adults (fall semester), or as part of a TB skin testing program. Discuss the collective experiences among all students near the end of the clinical laboratory course.

Evaluation Strategies

A. Multiple Choice Questions

1. The most frequently reported communicable disease in the United States is
   a. gonorrhea.
   b. syphilis.
   c. AIDS.
   d. tuberculosis.

2. HIV/AIDS present an intriguing and complex service delivery problem due to issues such as
   a. which of the curative treatments are best to use.
   b. sexual behaviors, illegal drug use and end-of-life issues.
   c. the highly vulnerable and risky position of caregivers.
   d. the negative attitude of HIV/AIDS clients toward caregivers.

3. There are three major goals to be achieved with the HIV-infected population. Which of the following is one of them?
   a. Achieving a speedy and comfortable death
   b. Minimizing the number of infections the HIV client acquires
   c. Locating housing options as the HIV clients' health deteriorates
   d. Delaying the onset of clinical symptoms with antiviral therapy

4. Tuberculosis Classification III means the person has
   a. what is called a TB infection.
   b. a positive skin test and chest x-ray.
   c. a less severe case of TB than those with class V.
   d. a less chance of getting TB than if they had class I or II.

5. Which of the following is an example of primary prevention and communicable disease control?
   a. Administering TB skin tests to 5 year old children entering kindergarten
   b. Providing chest x-rays to people with positive TB skin tests
   c. Performing the Western Blot test for HIV
   d. Administering immunizations to senior citizens at a flu clinic

B. True/False Questions

1. Approximately 20 percent of the worlds population is infected with Mycobacterium Tuberculosis.
   a. True
   b. False

2. A negative TB skin test in clients with AIDS means the client is free of TB.
   a. True
   b. False

3. Active immunity is a short term resistance to a specific disease-causing organism.
   a. True
   b. False

4. Non-compliance with the full TB treatment regimen has contributed to the development of drug-resistant strains.
   a. True
   b. False

5. TB kills one million people each year, worldwide.
   a. True
   b. False

C. Essay Questions

1. Express your thoughts in approximately 200 words by using the following introductory sentence "If I cared for an AIDS client in his/her home I would feel....."

2. In the United States the TB skin test (Mantoux, PPD) is used as the standard method for evaluating TB infection. In other countries the BCG vaccine is used routinely. Explain how you feel about each choice and give your rationale.

D. Individual or Group Projects

1. Assist in a survey of the entire population of a senior citizen housing unit receiving flu and pneumonia immunizations, either from a personal health care provider or flu clinic. Inquire into reasons for not receiving the vaccines. Are all medically eligible seniors receiving the vaccines? Why or why not? What can a community health nurse do about it?

2. Spend time with a school nurse as entering kindergarten children are assessed for immunization compliance. What barriers existed for families of underimmunized children? What percent were underimmunized or unimmunized? Discuss these issues with the school nurse and ask how he/she resolves the problems.

24 Promoting and Protecting the Health of At-Risk Populations

Learning Objectives

- Explain the concept of vulnerabilty and why some groups of people are at greater risk for health problems.
- Analyze each of the four causal domains contributing to vulnerability.
- Describe the etiology of the three types of homelessness.
- Discuss the health-related needs of the homeless population.
- Identify the factors from the four causal domains contributing to the problems of the mentally impaired population.
- Explain the causal factors and health-related problems of the substance abusing population.
- Discuss the community health nurses's role with at-risk populations.

Key Terms

- At-risk population
- Chemical addiction
- Chemical dependence
- Chronically homeless
- Depressants
- Episodically homeless
- Genetic predisposition
- Hallucinogens
- Homelessness
- Inhalants
- Marijuana
- Mentally impaired
- Narcotics
- Risk factors
- Steroids
- Stimulants
- Substance abuse
- Temporarily homeless
- Vulnerability

Chapter Summary

Chapter 24 looks at and explains the concept of vulnerability and why some groups of people are more at-risk for health problems than the general public. High-risk groups have always been a special challenge for the community health nurse. Selected at-risk populations are discussed in-depth in this chapter; the homeless, mentally impaired, and the substance abusing population.

Populations at-risk are vulnerable and several factors contribute to being vulnerable. These factors are derived from four general causal domains: biologic, behavioral, sociocultural, and environmental. Community health nurses have a crucial role to play among the multiple determinants of vulnerability. Nursing actions are suggested for each variable in each domain throughout this chapter.

The biologic domain has five variables that impact vulnerability: genetic predisposition, age, gender, race or ethnicity, and physical or mental impairment.

The behavioral domain includes lifestyle choices as variables, that in combination with each other or with those from other domains, place people at risk for health problems. These variables include diet and weight control, exercise and rest, emotional health and stress management, substance abuse and sexual practices.

The sociocultural domain presents additional variables of economic status and education, cultural values and practices, social support systems including spiritual health, and health care quality and access.

The final domain is environmental. Such variables as climate, geography and the home, work, and community are explored for potential effects on vulnerability.

Several specific at-risk populations are explored for their particular vulnerability to health problems. The first group discussed is the homeless. There are three types of homeless: the temporarily homeless, the episodically homeless, and the chronically homeless. Each group is homeless for very different reasons and the community health nurse approaches each group differently. There are many factors contributing to homelessness including physical and emotional illness, spousal abuse, poverty, unemployment and lack of affordable housing, substance abuse, poor stress management, and the deinstitutionalization of the mentally ill. All contribute to the problem of homelessness.

The needs of the homeless are great, especially the needs of the homeless with children. Women and children as a subgroup of homeless have been increasing in numbers and have a unique set of needs including infectious nuisance diseases, an interrupted educational process, and underimmunization. In addition they have the additional stress of finding shelter and assuring privacy for the family members in the homeless family with children. All of the homeless are vulnerable to stressors and emotional health problems caused by or accentuated by being homeless. Unfortunately, the health care delivery system provides services for the homeless mostly at the secondary and tertiary levels of prevention. Social policies will need to change to have prevention of homelessness a priority. Chapter 28 provides many suggestions for community health nurses involvement in the political arena, where change can occur.

The mentally-impaired population is the second at-risk group highlighted in this chapter. They have limited ability to function due to significant behavioral or psychological disorders. The exact number of mentally impaired is hard to estimate since it has not been a reportable condition. The National Institute of Mental Health has targeted three goals for this population: 1) to determine reliable incidence and prevalence of mental disorders, 2) to explore possible causes, and 3) to assist with planning and development of mental health services. The needs of this population are as varied as the types and severity of the mental disorders. Poor medication compliance, poor nutrition, emotional problems, and unstable housing are primary issues. These are summarized in Table 24-2. The community health nurse works best with this population in a community support system model. This model includes a comprehesive approach, with twelve distinct components, to support the mentally ill and disabled. Most services are secondary and tertiary in nature. Primary prevention needs to be enhanced and focused on. The community health nurse can work effectively in the community in this area of prevention.

The final vulnerable group covered in this chapter is the substance abusing population. The commonly abused substances fall into seven categories: cannabis, depressants, hallucinogens, inhalants, narcotics, steroids, and stimulants. Each category is reviewed and commonly abused substances within each category are mentioned. The etiology of substance abuse remains under study with no consensus about the causes. The behavioral/psychological causative factors are varied: peer pressure, family stress, low self-esteem, misleading information regarding over-the-counter drugs, over prescription of medications, and dysfunctional family systems. Much damage occurs from substance abuse. Serious health problems, psychological problems, and social problems are apparent in this population. The primary, secondary, and tertiary levels of prevention, and role of the community health nurse is covered and focuses on primary prevention. However, when the nurse encounters a substance abusing client there is a system of health care available and meeting the client's holistic needs is the essential goal.

Teaching Strategies

A. Classroom Strategies

1. Invite the director of a local homeless shelter to discuss some of the problems the homeless population encounters. Explore with the speaker what services the shelter offers in addition to temporary housing. You may want to obtain a speaker from a mental health center or a substance abuse program and discuss the same questions.

2. Place three columns on a transparency headed primary, secondary and tertiary prevention for homelessness. Have students suggest activities for each level of prevention to fill in the columns. Upon completion discuss the options suggested.

B. Clinical Laboratory Strategies

1. Explore the services offered by the American Red Cross to clients experiencing disasters (house fires, floods, tornados, etc.). If possible, spend some clinical laboratory hours assisting the disaster relief team from this agency.

2. Provide nursing services to a group of women with infants living in a drug rehabilitation home and plan to teach a health focused class on a topic such as: teaching the mothers how to make inexpensive toys for their children, providing anticipatory guidance and parenting skill information, or teaching the mothers games to play with their children which promote healthy parent/child interaction.

Evaluation Strategies

A. Multiple Choice Questions

1. Which of the following is a description of a client who is temporarily homeless?
   a. The client has been laid off from work for the third time this year
   b. A client's home has been destroyed by a tornado
   c. A client abuses alcohol and has no resources or marketable skills
   d. A client uses drugs and alcohol when there are too many stressors

2. Which of the following is a description of a client who is chronically homeless?
   a. The client has been laid off from work for the third time this year
   b. A client's home has been destroyed by a tornado
   c. A client abuses alcohol and has no resources or marketable skills
   d. A client uses drugs and alcohol when there are too many stressors

3. One of the goals of the National Institute of Mental Health involving the mentally impaired is
   a. treating all mentally impaired clients.
   b. eliminating mental impairment.
   c. promoting mental health in children.
   d. exploring causes of mental impairment.

4. An example of a behavioral factor influencing vulnerability to a mental disorder is
   a. anxiety over inadequate income.
   b. childhood neglect and abuse.
   c. birth defects and injuries at birth.
   d. living in excessively wet and gloomy weather.

5. A common characteristic of a drug dependent person is one who has
   a. self destructive tendencies.
   b. a low level of intelligence.
   c. an addiction to two or more drugs.
   d. over achievement in school activities.

B. True/False Questions

1. Ten percent of the homeless are mentally ill.
   a. True
   b. False

2. The four causal domains of vulnerability include biological, behavioral, sociocultural, and environmental.
   a. True
   b. False

3. A nursing action to eliminate environmental variables includes advocating for a healthier environment.
   a. True
   b. False

4. Less than one percent of substance abusers are chemically addicted.
   a. True
   b. False

5. Mothers with young children are the fastest growing group of homeless.
   a. True
   b. False

C. Essay Questions

1. Compare and contrast the three types of homeless people and identify the nurse's role with each group.

2. Describe the primary prevention methods that a community health nurse could use to promote the mental health of clients (children, teens, adults, or older adults). Select one age group and itemize your actions.

D. Individual or Group Projects

1. Meet with the director of a homeless shelter and discuss some specific needs of the shelter. Plan to meet one or some of those needs as an ongoing project throughout the clinical laboratory course. Some needs might be solved by a clothing drive, creation of a safe play area for children, preparation and serving of a holiday meal, or the planning of an immunization clinic at the shelter.

2. Have the clinical laboratory group of students locate a group of pregnant teens and have each student work with one teen to provide support, be an educational resource, be a counselor, advocate, and a friend. If the opportunity is available encourage the students to work with the teen over two or more semesters to provide continuity and to be a support during the pregnancy and during the first one to two years of the infant's life. (Possibly incorporate hours a student spends with the teen as part of another course's objectives.)

25

Leadership, Power, and Effecting Change in Community Health

Learning Objectives

- Describe the three characteristics of leadership.
- Summarize six leadership theories.
- Explain the difference between transformational and transactional leadership.
- Describe five leadership functions.
- Differentiate between four power bases and four power sources.
- Discuss the concept of empowerment and its significance for community health nursing.
- Explain the three stages of change.
- Discuss the eight steps in planned change.
- Identify three planned change strategies.
- Summarize six principles for effecting change in community health.

Key Terms

- Autocratic leadership style
- Autonomous leadership style
- Change
- Empirical-rational change strategy
- Empowerment
- Evolutionary change
- Force field analysis
- Leadership
- Normative-reeducative change strategy
- Participative leadership style
- Planned change
- Power

- Power bases
- Power-coercive change strategy
- Power sources
- Revolutionary change

- Stages of change
- Transactional leadership
- Transformational leadership

Chapter Summary

The role of the community health nurse as a leader and change agent is described in Chapter 25. Positively changing the health beliefs and improving the practices of individuals, families, and groups is a goal of community health nursing. As a leader, the community health nurse has power to effect change at the community level. The aim of a community health nurse's interaction in the community is to influence clients towards optimal health and to lead people to change also at the organizational level. In a leadership position in community or professional organizations, or as a member of a health planning board, the community health nurse is in a position of power. With this power comes the ability to influence others to make needed changes.

Leadership is described as a purposeful, interpersonal, and influential process that facilitates the accomplishment of a goal. Six theoretical approaches that give insight into the nature of leadership are discussed. They are trait theory, behavioral theory, contingency theory, leadership style theories, attribution theory, and charismatic theory. The history of the development of each theory category is presented with an overview of the theory. The leadership behavior grid (Figure 25-2, p. 580), the style of leadership chart (Figure 25-3, p. 581), and the leadership styles continuum (Figure 25-4, p. 582) depict some of the concepts of leadership theory. In addition to a theoretical basis to a leadership style there are two approaches leaders take with followers. A transactional leadership style encourages an exchange between leader and followers which clarifies roles and tasks to achieve goals. Transformational leadership is an approach that inspires followers to high levels of commitment and effort to achieve goals. Five functions are required for effective leadership at any level: 1) the creative function, 2) the initiating function, 3) the risk-taking function, 4) the integrative function, and 5) the instrumental function.

A community health nurse is in a leadership role because of the wide sphere of influence the role encompasses. The central aim of this leadership is to positively influence community health, and this is accomplished by influencing community leaders and agencies and their attitudes and programs. This sphere varies depending on the nurse's abilities, time available, work situation and the health care needs in the community. However, the ultimate test of nurse leadership is in the outcomes that come from effective leadership. Central to being effective is a relationship of trust, respect, and mutual exchange between leader and followers.

Power is the ability to influence or control other people's behaviors to accomplish desired goals. Power comes from five bases: 1) coercive power uses force to gain compliance, 2) reward power provides something of value in exchange for compliance, 3) expert power exerts influence by means of special knowledge and skills, 4) legitimate power derives from the person's position or title, and 5) referent power comes from others admiration and emulation of the powerholder. This information about power is not complete. Four types of power bases enable the powerholder to exert influence over others: information power, persuasive power, reward power, and coercive power. In addition, power sources come from four sources; from one's position, personal qualities, expertise, and opportunities. Community health nurses should develop their source of power and move into positions of influence in the health care delivery system.

Another task of the nurse in a leadership position is to be able to empower people so they can make changes in their own lives. The control over the decisions that affect one's life could enable all people, especially groups at-risk, to take charge and make healthy changes in their lives. For a vulnerable person or group to change and feel powerful instead of powerless and to make choices and be self determined takes the skillful leadership of a community health nurse. Achieving empowerment is germaine to effective leadership in the community.

As leaders, community health nurses are in a position to be the agent for change. Change can be viewed positively or negatively by those involved. According to Lippett (1973, p. 37), change is "any planned or unplanned alteration of the status quo in an organization, situation, or process." Change can be evolutionary or revolutionary. Evolutionary change evolves gradually in increments and does not require major adjustments or shifts in values or goals. It may be referred to as reform. Revolutionary change occurs suddenly, is more drastic and threatening, and requires people to adopt different values on radically new patterns of behavior. The process of change occurs in three stages, according to Lewin: unfreezing, changing, and refreezing. Unfreezing occurs when the need for change develops, creating disequilibrium in the system. The second stage occurs when a change is examined, accepted, and is tried. Refreezing takes place when the change is integrated and becomes a permanent part of the system.

Planned change can be described as a purposeful effort designed to effect improvement in a system with the assistance of a change agent. There are four characteristics key to successful change: the change must be purposeful and intentional; the change is by design, not default; it aims at improvement; and is accomplished by means of an influencing agent. The process of successfully managing change involves eight steps: 1) assess the symptoms, 2) diagnose needs, 3) analyze alternative solutions, 4) select change, 5) plan the change, 6) implement change, 7) evaluate change, and 8) stabilize change (see planned change model, Figure 25-7, p. 592).

Force-field analysis is a useful tool for the community health nurse implementing change. Examination of the restraining and driving forces for change will assist the nurse, as the change agent, to develop strategies to influence the forces for change (see Figure 25-8, p. 594).

Three different sets of strategies may be used singly or in combination to implement planned change: empirical-rational, normative-reeducative, and power-coercive. Empirical-rational strategies are based on the assumption that people are rational and when presented wth empirical data they will adopt changes that are in their best interest. Normative-reeducative strategies not only present new information, but directly influence the individual's attitudes and behaviors through persuasion. The use of coercion based on fear to bring about change is characteristic of the power-coercive strategy.

Six principles that serve as guidelines for effecting positive change are: 1) the principle of participation, 2) the principle of resistance to change, 3) the principle of proper timing, 4) the principle of interdependence, 5) the principle of flexibility, and 6) the principle of self-understanding.

Teaching Strategies

A. **Classroom Strategies**

1. Prior to the class on Chapter 25 content, have the students respond in writing to the following questions. (The responses should be confidential, but ask for volunteers to discuss their responses.)

   a. Who is the most effective person or best leader you have personally known?

   b. What are his/her major characteristics?

   c. Describe the worst leader you have ever personally known?

   d. What makes the leader so bad?

2. Think of a community health nurse who is an effective leader. Ask the nurse to speak to the class about situations he/she has encountered in his/her role as a leader and change agent.

B. **Clinical Laboratory Strategies**

1. Assign the students to identify forces that they would like to change. Ask the students to identify forces that may inhibit change and discuss how they, as change agents, would facilitate the change process.

2. Assign the students to interview a well-known community leader (mayor, religious leader, etc.). Questions the students might ask include the following:

   a. What are your present concerns for the community?

   b. What are your visions for the future?

   c. How do you view your role as a community leader?

   d. What obstacles have you encountered acting as a change agent?

   e. How would you describe your leadership style?

Evaluation Strategies

A. Multiple Choice Questions

1. What are Lewin's three stages of change?
   a. Unfreezing, planning, and integrating
   b. Unlearning, learning, and relearning
   c. Planning, organizing, and coordinating
   d. Unfreezing, changing, and refreezing

2. The normative-reeducative strategy of change assumes that
   a. people are rational and will adopt a new practice because it is in their best interest.
   b. compliance by the client system will occur through the use of power to effect change.
   c. information alone is not enough, and behaviors change through persuasion.

3. Autocratic leadership style
   a. uses the power of the position to influence followers.
   b. involves followers in the decision-making process.
   c. is facilitative and encourages independence among group members.
   d. encourages the use of magnetic and inspirational personality and behaviors.

4. Participative leadership style
   a. uses the power of the position to influence followers.
   b. involves followers in the decision-making process.
   c. is facilitative and encourages independence among group members.
   d. encourages the use of magnetic and inspirational personality and behaviors.

5. Reward power influences others by
   a. providing something of value in exchange for compliance.
   b. means of special knowledge or skills.
   c. the legitimate power that comes with the title or position.
   d. using force to gain compliance.

B. True/False Questions

1. Evolutionary change tends to occur rapidly and may upset the balance of things system.
   a. True
   b. False

2. Leaders should not be risk takers, they need to proceed under sure conditions.
   a. True
   b. False

3. Community health nurses can and should positively influence the community's health.
   a. True
   b. False

4. Unfreezing is the first stage of a three step change model.
   a. True
   b. False

5. Planned change is purposeful and intentional.
   a. True
   b. False

C. Essay Questions

1. Describe the attributes an ideal leader should have in the role of Director of Nursing in a community agency.

2. Briefly describe your leadership style. What aspects of your style would you like to change?

D. Group/Individual Projects

1. Perhaps several students are working on a group project in some class they are taking. Suggest they examine the leadership style of the group leader. Have the students answer the following questions: What did the leader do right and wrong? What leadership style did they display? How would you have lead the group differently?

2. Complete a group project using the Activities to Promote Critical Thinking at the end of Chapter 25.

26

Research in Community Health Nursing

Learning Objectives

- Explain the difference between quantitative research and qualitative research.
- Describe the eight steps of the research process.
- Differentiate between experimental and nonexperimental research design.
- Analyze the potential impact of research on community health nursing practice.
- Identify the community health nurse's role in conducting research and using research findings.

Key Terms

- Conceptual model
- Control group
- Descriptive statistics
- Experimental design
- Experimental group
- Generalizability
- Inferential statistics
- Instrument
- Nonexperimental design
- Qualitative research
- Quantitative research
- Randomization
- Reliability
- Research
- Validity

Chapter Summary

Research has an important place within community health nursing. In order to serve the health needs of communities, nurses need to be familiar with the boundaries, characteristics, and specific health risks of client populations. By conducting research projects nurses can examine topics of interest and add to the body of nursing knowledge, thereby promoting the health level of at-risk populations.

Nursing research is approached by one of two methodologies: quantitative research or qualitative research. Quantitative research collects data that can be measured objectively and usually focuses on parts rather than on the whole. Qualitative research is more subjective and is the preferred method when a broader focus is needed. Both approaches are rigorous and systematic, although the design and purpose is different.

The process of conducting effective research follows a series of specific steps: 1) identify an area of interest, 2) formulate a research question or statement, 3) review the literature, 4) select a conceptual model, 5) choose a research design, 6) collect and analyze data, 7) interpret the results, and 8) communicate findings. Each step of the research process is described in this chapter, and examples of published community health nursing research topics are presented.

Areas of research interest for community health nurses include disease prevention, wellness, and the active involvement of clients in their care. These topics provide the nurse investigator with a broad research selection that will have an impact on the community or facilitate an improvement in health states of individuals, groups, and communities.

The nurse investigator must narrow the topic to a researchable question that is achievable and within the resources available. A clearly stated research question provides direction for the investigator. The next step of the research process is a review of the existing literature. During the first phase the researcher scans available publications to develop a superficial knowledge about the area of interest to determine the value of pursuing a given topic. The second phase involves an in-depth critical search of all publications relevant to the topic of interest. The literature should be current, relevant, and from primary or secondary sources. A well formulated research question identifies: 1) the population of interest, 2) the variable or variables to be measured, and 3) the interventions (if used).

Selection of a conceptual model for the research topic will help to clarify the focus and direction of the study and the interpretation of the findings. The advantage of using nursing models is that they provide an understanding of the world in terms of nursing's major concerns.

An experimental research design is characterized by manipulation of a variable, randomization of subjects, and use of a control group. Nonexperimental designs, in which the nurse describes existing relationships or observed behavior, often lay the groundwork for experiments. In many cases a true experimental study is difficult, or even impossible to conduct, so the nurse must conduct quasi-experimental research. Quasi-experimental research designs lack either randomization of subjects or designation of a control group.

A variety of data collection methods are presented in this chapter: questionnaires, observation guides, assessments, and diaries. Instruments used are evaluated for accuracy using validity and reliability tests. Descriptive statistics describe the data collected, and inferential statistics imply that the findings from the research sample are likely to exist in a larger population. Research findings determine the validity of the hypothesis of the study.

Interpretation of the results should make sense in relationship to the conceptual model, review of literature, and methodology (data collection methods). Findings from studies give future nurse researchers direction. An important function of conducting research is to contribute to building the nursing knowledge that can be applied to improve care to clients. The final step of the research process is communication of the results. Little benefit will be derived from an investigation if the results are not shared with appropriate others.

Research in the community health area has the potential to have a significant impact on: 1) public policy and the community's health, 2) the effectiveness of community health nursing practice, and 3) the status and influence of nursing as a profession. Community health nurses have two important responsibilities in respect to research in community health: 1) to apply the research findings and 2) to conduct nursing research. By keeping current with research in community health, findings can be applied to the practice setting. Finally, there is a need for more community health nurses to conduct research themselves or in collaboration with a team of health care workers in the community.

Teaching Strategies

A. Classroom Strategies

1. Arrange for nurses who are working in the community, or at the university and participating in research, to speak to the class about their research activities. Encourage them to discuss both successes and pitfalls associated with their efforts.

2. Assign students to bring to class community health nursing research articles from current (within the last five years) journals. Each student should select or be assigned a specific topic of interest (such as AIDS, stress reduction, battered spouses, or health promotion). Use the journal articles to discuss the steps of the

research process and the role of the community health nurse in conducting research.

B. Clinical Laboratory Strategies

1. Have the students identify an area of interest specific to their clinical laboratory setting that could be the focus of a community health nursing investigation. At a clinical conference ask the students to describe how an investigation could be conducted and what impact such a study would have on community health nursing practice. Recommend that students share their research ideas with the clinical staff, if appropriate.

2. Ask the students to discuss with agency personnel research activities in which these individuals are participating, or have participated, and their plans for future study. Have students share this information during a clinical conference or in their clinical laboratory journals.

Evaluation Strategies

A. Multiple Choice Questions

1. The function of a conceptual model for a research study is to
   a. clarify the focus and direction of the study.
   b. provide evidence that an instrument is valid.
   c. limit the breadth and depth of the study.
   d. enhance the adaptability of findings to other disciplines.

2. Inferential statistics may be used to analyze data. This form of statistical analysis
   a. infers that the data collected is appropriate for the conceptual model.
   b. implies that relationships found in the group studied can be generalized to a larger group.
   c. permits the investigator to initiate a preliminary investigation of subjects.
   d. describes the data collected in an organized manner according to defined variables.

3. An experimental design requires that the investigator
   a. manipulate one of the variables.
   b. non-randomly assign subjects to groups.
   c. control all variables without manipulation.
   d. balance the study with four study groups.

4. The literature review for a research study includes which of the following?
   a. An in-depth study of the literature in the area of interest for at least the last twenty years
   b. An overview of current literature in the area followed by an in-depth study of literature in the last five years
   c. Multiple sources of information including current lay literature, historic documents, and the tabloid press
   d. No more than three to five articles that are studied in-depth and incorporated into the body of the study

5. A variety of data collection sources are used by nurse researchers and include
   a. gossip.
   b. hearsay.
   c. opinion.
   d. rumors.

B. True/False Questions

1. Nursing research studies should be done by one nurse investigator to keep them ideally focused.
   a. True
   b. False

2. There are three steps in the research process that must be followed, the others are arbitrary.
   a. True
   b. False

3. Qualitative research is not as valuable as quantitative research.
   a. True
   b. False

4. Experimental studies can be expensive and hard to conduct.
   a. True
   b. False

5. It is important to determine the validity and reliability of data collection tools before using them.
   a. True
   b. False

C. Essay Questions

1. Think of the disease process or health related issue affecting the last community health client you visited. Using the steps of the research process design a study involving that issue. Describe a study that could be conducted in your community with resources you know are available.

2. Follow the same format suggested in question #1, but select a health related issue that you see in yourself (stress, weight, organization, spirituality, etc.) and design a study with students in nursing as the subjects.

D. Individual/Group Projects

1. Suggest to the employees or administration in an agency with which you are affiliated, that one or several students assist them in conducting research. As a part of the course requirements, actively include yourself in the research process.

2. Assist a faculty member in current research he or she is conducting. All steps of the research process are appropriate for student involvement. However, the research steps that are especially suited for student involvement are the literature review, data collection, and communicating the findings.

Quality Management in Community Health Nursing

Learning Objectives

- Define quality care.
- Discuss the historical development of quality care attainment in the delivery of community health care.
- Compare and contrast the four models of quality management in community health care.
- Identify the three primary areas of focus in a quality management program.
- Identify the six characteristics of quality community health programs.
- Describe how quality care is assessed and measured.
- Discuss the role of the nurse in a quality management program in a community health care setting.

Key Terms

- Audit
- Concurrent review
- Peer review
- Quality assurance
- Quality care
- Quality circles
- Quality control
- Quality indicators
- Retrospective review
- Standards for care
- Total quality management

Chapter Summary

Quality management, as a comprehensive term, includes all the activities an agency undertakes to assure that the highest quality of service is delivered, by qualified practitioners, in a well organized system of delivery, at a cost that keeps the program viable. Although quality care delivery is only a part of the quality management picture, it is the most important part, and the one on which nurses most traditionally have focused. In today's environment of cost containment and managed care, the broader picture of quality management must be the focus.

Historically, nursing has evolved over the years as a self regulating profession from three perspectives: 1) clinical competence, 2) organizational competence, and 3) a nursing care review process. Standardized basic and advanced education for nurses is assured by state regulation and accrediting bodies. Licensure and certification of nurses in all states, along with continuing education requirements, determines competence. Since the 1940s institutions have been monitored for the quality of the services they deliver. These regulations have become more stringent in recent years. There are now many more agencies delivering a variety of health care services than ever before. Competition for clients demands that the highest standards be met by the agency and its employees if the agency wishes to remain in business. Today's consumer is knowledgeable and demands a high level of service.

The evolution of health care delivery and economics places agencies in a position to incorporate a model for quality management. Four specific models are shared in Chapter 27 as examples of tested systems in the health care arena. The Donabedian model, the ANA model, the Upwardly spiraling feedback loop model, and the Hoesing and Kirk quality management models are discussed.

The Donabedian model looks at the structure (facility resources), process (standards and attitudes), and outcome (client health care goals) of quality and is often the framework for more complex models. The American Nurses Association (ANA) provides a quality improvement model that uses the Donabedian model and is based on standards of care and quality indicators. The Upwardly spiraling feedback loop model takes the ANA model a bit further and adds a feedback loop, making the process dynamic, so change can occur in response to ongoing feedback. The forth model developed by Hoesing and Kirk (1990) focuses on the "big picture" and provides the clarity needed to manage quality and to monitor and evaluate results. The model is designed for supervisory and administrative personnel as well as for the individual professional nurse.

Quality management is an important component of community health nursing. Serving the health care needs of populations requires that limited resources be put to the most effective use. Agencies use several quality management strategies that assess quality care in the community and become a part of the way to deliver services. Audit tools such as record review, checklists, questionnaires, and surveys provide the feedback quality review or audit committees need to make decisions about future care. Involving the professional staff in a quality circle (a form of participative management used in successful businesses in Japan for forty years) increases employee responsibility for decision making and problem solving. Other tools, such as measuring client outcomes through the quantitative measurement of quality indicators, define and quantify outcomes of care and greatly assist the staff in evaluating the results of care provided.

Quality management in community health nursing assists agencies (with limited resources and escalating costs) to determine what programs are effective and best serve the needs of the community. There are six characteristics considered essential in the development and maintenance of quality community health programs, that it: 1) addresses the interrelated health needs of the entire person or community, and is comprehensive 2) demonstrates organizational competency, is expertly managed and financially sound, 3) demonstrates professional competency and a commitment to personal excellence among a competent staff, 4) is accessible and has services readily available to its clients in a timely manner despite barriers that may exist, 5) is efficient and makes the best use of resources, and 6) demonstrates its consideration of client priorities and positive effects of the health status on clients as measured by client outcomes, thus increasing the client's interest to return to the same agency when services are needed again.

The community health nurse manages the quality of care delivered within the community. Through the framework of structure, process, and outcomes, the nurse working in a community agency has a role to assume. The organizational structure remains client focused with sufficient resources, and a system of acquiring additional funding, to maintain present services and to offer new services as needed. Services are delivered to a growing number of clients by a highly motivated and qualified staff. The process is monitored by staff contributing to continuous and ongoing evaluation of standards. Staff work collaboratively and are supported by administration with job skills requirements updated as needed. The client outcomes, based on standards of care, are met or surpassed and are consistent with agency goals and quality care.

Teaching Strategies

A. Classroom Strategies

1. Ask a representative of a health care agency in the community to speak to the class about the process of quality management used in the agency. What specific quality assurance tools do they use? How do the nurses in the agency participate in the quality management program?

2. Examine the four models of quality management presented in this chapter and determine the one(s) most helpful for a public agency (city health department) and private agency (a for-profit home health agency). Discuss reasons for the decisions made.

B. Clinical Laboratory Strategies

1. In the agency in which students are having their clinical laboratory practicum, ask one of the nursing administrators to discuss the agency's quality management system for nursing.
2. Have the students conduct a chart audit on a client they are serving, using the agency's quality management assessment tools (checklist, survey, etc.).

Evaluation Strategies

A. Multiple Choice Questions

1. Facilitation of ongoing self-evaluation is accomplished through
   a. standard measurement.
   b. the nursing process.
   c. quality indicators.
   d. management by objectives.

2. The six dimensions of a quality health care program are comprehensiveness, effectiveness, acceptability, accessibility, efficiency, and provider competence. In evaluating **accessibility**, which of the following questions would be appropriate?
   a. Does the agency connect with the population served and find adequate ways to meet the public's health needs?
   b. Do the services provided make use of available funds?
   c. Are the nurses using the most current information and resources available?
   d. Is the population being served satisfied with the care and functioning at a higher level as a result of that care?

3. The six dimensions of a quality health care program are comprehensiveness, effectiveness, acceptability, accessibility, efficiency, and provider competence. In evaluating **efficiency**, which of the following questions would be appropriate?

    a. Does the agency connect with the population served and find adequate ways to meet the public's health needs?

    b. Do the services provided make use of available funds?

    c. Are the nurses using the most current information and resources available?

    d. Is the population being served satisfied with the care and functioning at a higher level as a result of that care?

4. Health care goals that can be used to evaluate structure, process, and outcome of care are known as

    a. criteria.

    b. process data.

    c. evaluation issues.

    d. standards.

5. A quality circle can best be described as

    a. the financing of an organization from purchasing through to delivery.

    b. the parameters a nurse must consider as care is delivered.

    c. a style of participative management that shares the decision-making process with staff.

    d. a form of reward to an agency when they have met criteria demonstrating excellence.

B. True/False Questions

1. The Donabedian model for quality management looks at assessment, problem identification, and action.

    a. True

    b. False

2. The four models of quality management presented in Chapter 27 are based on the concepts of structure, process, and outcome.

    a. True

    b. False

3. Quality management should be built into an agency through all aspects of its functioning.
   a. True
   b. False

4. Quality indicators are quality-focused objectives used as markers to determine whether a goal has been met.
   a. True
   b. False

5. Retrospective review of a client's chart occurs while care is still being delivered to them.
   a. True
   b. False

C. Essay Questions

1. Review the charting you have done on a client you have been visiting. How would you be able to measure whether quality care had been delivered to this client by reviewing your charting?

2. Identify the services that you feel should be provided by the "ideal" community health agency. Using the six criteria for quality health care delivery outlined in Chapter 27, how would you measure success?

D. Individual/Group Projects

1. Ask the nurse manager of a community agency if you may participate in the chart audit process of the agency. Critique the methods used. Ask questions about the process and possibly make suggestions to improve the process in a meeting with the nursing manager.

2. Initiate a quality circle concept among a group of peers and your instructor in community health nursing. Use this participative management tool to evaluate the class functioning based on established standards (the course objectives).

28

Health Policy, Politics, and Community Health Advocacy

Learning Objectives

- Define health policy and explain how it is established.
- Analyze the influence of health policy on community health and nursing practice.
- Explain the role of special interest groups in health care reform and policy making.
- Identify the four stages in the policy process and briefly explain what each entails.
- Define political empowerment and describe ways in which community health nurses can become politically empowered.
- Explain the role of community health nurses in determining a community's health policy needs.
- Identify the ten steps in mobilizing a community for political action.
- Describe the steps involved in how a bill becomes a law.
- Explain several methods of communicating with legislators on policy issues.
- List at least four political strategies for community health nursing.

Key Terms

- Community health advocacy
- Distributive health policy
- Health policy
- Health policy outcomes
- Lobbying
- Polarization
- Policy

- Policy analysis
- Policy system
- Political action
- Political action committee (PAC)
- Political empowerment

- Politics
- Public policy
- Regulatory health policy
- Special interest group

Chapter Summary

Chapter 28 examines health policy, the political process involved in determining health policy, and the community health nurse's role in the process. Community health nurses should not only provide input to policy decision makers, but should be leaders who are in decision making situations. This chapter discusses the community health nurse's role and power in providing essential influence and a unique perspective in meeting health care needs.

Policy is an authoritatively stated course of action that guides the making of decisions. Health policy is about health care choices and, as in policy decisions in all arenas, the decisions made are often influenced by the stakeholders (anyone with a vested interest). Decisions at the federal or state levels lead to the formulation and implementation of health policy at a local level. Health policy should empower the community, but it also empowers the health care provider and often there are conflicts between the two.

Health policy is influenced by the collective power of various people known as special interest groups. Most often these collective voices have persuasive power to bow health policy in their favor. This may not always be in the best interest of the population as a whole. The four most powerful interest groups in health care have been physicians, hospitals, insurance companies, and the drug industry.

Nursing has become a stronger political voice in recent years and is learning to build alliances and power bases. Because the health care system is complex and represents many different interests, nursing has a challenge to make its interests heard. Health policy problems nurses face include delivering services that are not reimbursable and scope of practice.

The country is on the verge of major health care reform, and community health nurses deliver the services considered essential to these changes. This puts community health nurses in a position of power that needs to be recognized and acted upon. This can be done through the organized efforts of professional organizations. A short history of the need for, and interest in, policy reform is discussed.

Understanding policy systems and the analysis of policies is necessary in order to effect the system. Figure 28-3 provides a model for studying health policy. The four stages of policy adoption are: 1) formulation, 2) adoption, 3) implementation, and 4) evaluation.

Community health advocacy, or efforts aimed at creating awareness of, and generating support for, meeting the community's health needs, is an important role that community health nurses must assume. This can cause change at the community level. Nurses serve as facilitators in assessing the community's needs in relation to existing health care policies. Once this recognition is made, the community can organize for political action under the leadership of the community health nurse. This involves ten steps: 1) identifying yourself as a community organizer, 2) identifying problems, concerns, and issues; 3) assess the physical community, 4) assess community strengths, resources, and interests; 5) assess political influences in the community, 6) evaluate alternative courses of action, 7) redefine objectives, priorities, and the community health nurse's goals; 8) develop a plan of action, 9) implement the plan, and 10) evaluate the outcome of the planned action.

After following the ten steps to organizing political action, the change suggested is ready for acceptance through the legislative process so the change can become policy. The community health nurse needs to know how a bill becomes law. The step by step process of a proposal (bill) presented to the legislature (through committees, the Senate, House of Representatives, and the President) is discussed, as the bill makes its way to becoming law or policy. The beginning of the political process is at the grass-roots level with a political strategy. Community health nurses and nurses in general have not used their power at the local level to begin the process of change. Their integral role and responsibilities in the health care system have not been exerted. This starts by presenting a unified professional influence, improving individual and collective self-concept, learning to be personally and politically assertive, recognizing and respecting colleagues, and achieving a greater financial base to support the cost of having their political voice heard.

Individual guidelines for political involvement are shared in this chapter. There are actions to take to generate support for yourself, to generate legitimacy, and to resolve conflicts that may arise. Political involvement also includes communicating with public officials. Suggestions for written communication (including addressing and formulating a letter), personal visits, and attending hearings and providing testimony are included.

Teaching Strategies

A. Classroom Strategies

1. Invite a community activist to speak to the class about his/her area of political interest if it affects existing health policies. If possible, find a community health nurse who is involved in these issues.

2. Have students analyze a policy on a health issue affecting the local community. Find out who benefits and who loses as a result of the policy. Use the policy

analysis model in Figure 28-3, p. 643. Follow-up on views by writing a letter to a political leader in regard to the policy analyzed.

B. **Clinical Laboratory Strategies**

1. Have students attend a city council or board of supervisors meeting in their local community. In a clinical conference share the community health related policies under discussion at the meeting and determine how the policies came about and if they need to be changed.

2. Have students complete a community survey. They should determine the gaps in health service that are of concern to the community, find out who the most active people are in this area of concern, and learn what is being done to alleviate the problem(s).

Evaluation Strategies

A. **Multiple Choice Questions**

1. Health policy should
   a. reflect a community's values.
   b. be made for a few influential people.
   c. be created by people outside of the community.
   d. reflect the needs of the community's poor.

2. An example of a regulatory health policy is
   a. federal subsidy for nursing education.
   b. benefits for needy groups.
   c. licensure of health professionals.
   d. allocating resources among groups.

3. The most troubling issue in health care that outweighs all others is
   a. accessibility.
   b. cost.
   c. quality of care.
   d. the uninsured.

4. The legislative process is
   a. a simple process designed for anyone to follow.
   b. a process that takes about three months.
   c. similar at the state and federal levels.
   d. initiated by the president of the United States.

5. Why is it important for community health nurses to understand the legislative process?
   a. The nurse may decide to add the role of political activist to the nursing role description
   b. Nurses need to become watchdogs of the activities of state and federal legislators
   c. The nurse's change agent role includes involvement in the community's political arena
   d. Legislative knowledge allows the nurse to be in control of health policy in the state

B. True/False Questions

1. Policy decisions are most often influenced by the stakeholders.
   a. True
   b. False

2. Health policies are made at the local level and affect state and federal levels.
   a. True
   b. False

3. Health policies are not influenced by special interest groups.
   a. True
   b. False

4. The stages of policy adoption include formulation, adoption, implementation, and evaluation.
   a. True
   b. False

5. The beginning of the political process can begin at the grass-roots level and effect major changes.
   a. True
   b. False

C. Essay Questions

1. When you consider the concept of health care reform, what changes do you envision and how will those changes be paid for?

2. Think of your political involvement thus far in your life (working for political candidates, writing letters to legislators, membership in a student nurse organization, etc.). How will that history affect your political involvement as a registered nurse?

D. Individual/Group Projects

1. Select an issue currently before your local, state or federal legislature and follow the progress of this issue (bill) throughout the semester. At the end of the semester report to the class as to the status of the bill. You may want to involve the class by having class members write letters to legislators.

2. Attend all local meetings or hearings on an issue of concern to you and your community. Present testimony from your perspective as a student in community health nursing and follow the steps outlined in Chapter 28 for generating support when becoming politically involved.

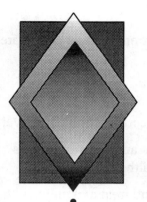

Answers to Evaluation Strategies

Chapter 1

Multiple-Choice Questions

1. b **Rationale**: A community of solution is represented by a group of people with solutions to a problem that affects them all and may come from a variety of geographic communities.

2. d **Rationale**: Involves actions at the tertiary level of prevention with persons, or communities, with disabilities or damage where restoration is needed.

3. b **Rationale**: Secondary prevention attempts to detect and treat existing health problems. Scoliosis most often occurs during adolescence when there is an accelerated growth rate. Early detection and treatment can prevent permanent structural changes.

4. c **Rationale**: Tertiary prevention seeks to reduce the extent and severity of a health problem. Parents of an infant who has died of SIDS have experienced a severe loss that will have an impact on their health and family functioning. Support groups such as those for parents of SIDS infants use tertiary prevention to lessen the impact on family members' lives.

5. c **Rationale**: Primary prevention involves anticipatory planning and action on the part of community health professionals. Community health nurses and local health departments need to envision potential needs and/or

problems so that they can design programs, or take action, to meet anticipated needs or prevent problems from occurring.

True/False Questions

1. a **Rationale**: Health and wellness can be measured subjectively and objectively.

2. a **Rationale**: Raising the level of wellness in individuals and communities is one of three health promotion goals in community health practice.

3. b **Rationale**: Secondary prevention attempts to detect and treat existing health problems as early as possible. Blood pressure screening is a way to detect hypertension in people who may not be diagnosed early in the disease since it often goes unrecognized by the client.

4. b **Rationale**: A group of student nurses is a common interest community. They may live in very diverse geographic communities.

5. a **Rationale**: Communities and populations are types of aggregates - the focus of community health practices.

Chapter 2

Multiple-Choice Questions

1. a **Rationale**: Official or public health care agencies are supported by tax dollars. They are also mandated to provide certain services because tax dollars support them.

2. d **Rationale**: Direct services are provided at the local level. The other levels guide, help finance, do research and generally support the local level.

3. b **Rationale**: Records are dated as early as 3000 B.C.. There are no written records of health care actions prior to this time.

4. d **Rationale**: At the height of the industrial revolution citizens finally accepted organized health care efforts. This occurred in the 1800s. Before that there was little or no organized health care services that lasted.

5. b **Rationale**: Voluntary agencies are funded by private donations. No federal mandates determine the services they provide.

True/False Questions

1. b **Rationale**: Progress is contributed to the efforts of Lemuel Shattuck. C. Everett Koop was the Surgeon General in the 1980s.

2. a **Rationale**: These are the core functions of public health services and are clearly discussed in Chapter 2.

3. a **Rationale**: Voluntary agencies are supported by private funding while official agencies are tax supported. These are the foundational differences between the two types of agencies.

4. b **Rationale**: There have been more than twenty significant pieces of health related legislation in the past seventy years.

5. a **Rationale**: The change to a prospective payment system through Diagnostic Related Groupings (DRGs) was initiated to halt rising health costs.

Chapter 3

Multiple-Choice Questions

1. a **Rationale**: HMOs are a prospective pay system and have existed since the 1930s. Paperwork for the client is minimal and simpler for the HMO. 15% of the population is enrolled in HMOs.

2. d **Rationale**: It is a federal health insurance program for the elderly. It covers less than half of health care costs for the elderly and only part B has a fee. 13% of the population is covered by Medicare.

3. b **Rationale**: The program is financed by federal and state monies, but administered by each state. It covers preventative services and has no cost to the truly indigent (in some states there is cost-sharing that fluctuates in amount).

4. c **Rationale**: NHI in some form is desired by the U.S. but has not yet been adopted. It is being discussed to cover everyone. It has been debated for almost a century, since 1912.

5. c **Rationale**: Health care economics needs to be understood by all nurses regardless of agency, position, or title. The future of a viable health care delivery depends on it.

True/False Questions

1. a **Rationale**: This payment system helps make HMOs cost effective and viable alternative health care delivery methods.

2. b **Rationale**: Historically this has not been true and contributes to the gap in public and private health care services. However, this does need to change.

3. a **Rationale**: They are single public sector insurers. They do not go through the 1500 insurance companies in the U.S..

4. b **Rationale**: This is happening. Some states are following this model. Oregon is one that is being looked at by other states considering adopting a similar model.

5. b **Rationale**: Prospective payment systems contribute to cost containment, eliminating incentives to provide more care. Retrospective systems contribute to rising health care costs.

Chapter 4

Multiple-Choice Questions

1. b **Rationale**: The numbers, variety of settings, and many other nurses coming to work in these community settings since the 1970s, has made the most significant difference. Politics, associations, or physicians made no significant impact in this change.

2. c **Rationale**: Phoebe is mentioned in the Bible as providing care to people in their home. The other names have no know significance to the history of early home care.

3. a **Rationale**: There are 6 identified characteristics of community health nursing. A focus on wellness is one of them. The other terms are not mentioned. Independence and care to groups would be more correct than dependence or individualism.

4. c **Rationale**: Orem's model focuses on self-care. The other models have different foci but are applicable to community health nursing for other reasons.

5. d **Rationale**: Homeostasis is a foundation of systems theories. This is the state of equilibrium between interacting parts of a whole. All organisms adapt to achieve homeostasis.

True/False Questions

1. b **Rationale**: Stressors are the internal or external forces that impact the health of people. In the community the focus is often on environmental stressors.

2. a **Rationale**: The basis of Orem's model is to promote independence and self-care in all clients. This speaks to the educator role of the community health nurse with an ambulatory population.

3. a **Rationale**: These are the four foundational concepts of Rogers' model.

4. a   **Rationale**: In Pender's model, people move to a healthier state they are more apt to practice healthy living behaviors, which will continue to move them to a higher state of wellness.

5. b   **Rationale**: In this model Roy proposes that adaptation levels fluctuate, and are constantly changing, due to many variables in people's lives.

Chapter 5

Multiple-Choice Questions

1. c   **Rationale**: Collecting data is one of the steps in the research process. This is the role most clearly identified.

2. a   **Rationale**: Working with a variety of colleagues to benefit client care is an example of the role of collaborator.

3. b   **Rationale**: Leading, or in effect teaching, in a childbirth preparation program demonstrates the role of educator.

4. d   **Rationale**: These are examples of the role of clinician: observing, listening, counseling and providing physical care.

5. a   **Rationale**: These activities demonstrate how the community health nurse manages her day by using the management functions of planning, organizing, leading and controlling/evaluating.

True/False Questions

1. a   **Rationale**: The goals of advocacy are to help clients gain greater independence and to make the system more responsive and relevant to their needs.

2. b   **Rationale**: Community health nursing practice is not limited to a specific arena - it can be practiced anywhere.

3. a   **Rationale**: Research is an investigative process, and from that perspective all community health nurses are researchers.

4. b   **Rationale**: The role of leader is distinguished from that of manager. As leaders, nurses influence, persuade, and act as change agents.

5. a   **Rationale**: To collaborate means to work jointly with others in a common endeavor, to cooperate as partners.

Chapter 6

Multiple-Choice Questions

1. d **Rationale**: The total relationship or patterns of relationships between people and their environment is known as the ecological perspective.

2. a **Rationale**: A vector is a nonhuman carrier of disease organisms that can transmit these organisms directly to humans.

3. d **Rationale**: Water pollution is not new and is a problem in all water sources in the United States, as well as other countries. It causes millions of cases of diseases yearly, some mild and some severe enough to cause death.

4. a **Rationale**: The EPA was established to have authority over all matters regarding the protection of public health.

5. b **Rationale**: Diapers are estimated to resist deterioration up to five centuries after burial in a landfill (Nadakavukaren, 1990). 18 billion diapers make up 2% of municipal waste and 99% of the people throw diapers away without flushing them first.

True/False Questions

1. a **Rationale**: Radon gas exposure has existed for many years especially in homes with cracked basements or built on dirt with deteriorating rocks in the soil. However, only recently has it become a topic of environmental concern.

2. b **Rationale**: Ground water has less contaminants than surface water but may still be unsafe due to runoff from agricultural pesticides and industrial wastes leaking into the ground.

3. b **Rationale**: There are 5 million cases of salmonella (from food sources) in the United States each year (Beneson, 1990).

4. a **Rationale**: This is the proper term for the role they play in environmental health.

5. a **Rationale**: There are 3000-3500 pounds of personal and industrial waste occurring per person per year in the United States (Moeller, 1992).

Chapter 7

Multiple Choice Questions

1. b **Rationale**: This group makes up 12% of the total population. The other groups make up 9, 3 and less than 1% of the population, respectively.

2. c **Rationale**: The Hispanic-American group is growing and will be 21% of the population by 2050, with the other groups representing 10, 15 and less than 1% of the population, respectively.

3. a **Rationale**: Being present oriented is a behavior of the culture of poverty. Usually it takes so much energy to meet the needs of today (food, shelter, clothing) that they have difficulty balancing thoughts in the past, present, and the future.

4. d **Rationale**: Native American similarities are shared in Table 7-1, p. 154. They live in the present, use traditional medicines, and value cooperation, in addition to valuing elders.

5. b **Rationale**: A person with a disability is seen as different; not deficient, abnormal or negative. (see Table 7-2, p. 161).

True/False Questions

1. b **Rationale**: It is the view that one's own culture is best, right and the only way of living, not valuing other cultural groups.

2. a **Rationale**: Cultures are always changing, adding and taking away parts that are not useful.

3. a **Rationale**: A subculture is a relatively large aggregate who share commonalities of geography, age, ethnicity, and so forth.

4. b **Rationale**: This is not a major disease among Asian/Pacific Rim-Americans. However, it is among African-Americans and Native Americans.

5. a **Rationale**: North Americans require a greater talking distance than Latin Americans, who are comfortable with an 18 inch talking distance.

Chapter 8

Multiple-Choice Questions

1. b **Rationale**: Prescriptive-proscriptive beliefs determine whether an action is desirable or undesirable. Moral evaluations are prescriptive-proscriptive beliefs.

2. a **Rationale**: Endurance provides continuity and stability to personal and social existence.

3. c **Rationale**: Equity is defined as the value directing like cases to be treated alike, and that all individuals be treated fairly.

4. a **Rationale**: Self-determination promotes individual autonomy and enhances self-concept, health-promoting behaviors, and quality of care.

5. c **Rationale**: The ANA Code is a guideline to follow as one practices nursing ethically. It is not a mandate, has no jurisdiction over licensure, nor does it make moral judgments.

True/False Questions

1. a **Rationale**: The discovery of one's values and the underlying motivations that guide one's actions is the purpose of values clarification.

2. b **Rationale**: The valuing process is a series of steps by which values become part of a person's belief system.

3. a **Rationale**: Values clarification can be used to analyze and understand how values are meaningful to people and ultimately influence their choices and behavior.

4. a **Rationale**: Evaluative judgments are statements of value, rights, duties, and responsibilities. Among the words to look for are want, desire, refer, should, ought, benefit, harm, duty, responsibility, right, or obligation.

5. b **Rationale**: When judgments involve moral values, conflicts are inevitable as the differences in moral values and beliefs clash.

Chapter 9

Multiple-choice questions

1. c **Rationale**: Community health nurses work at all levels of practice, and a prime mission is working with communities.

2. b **Rationale**: The problem-oriented assessment is commonly used when familiarization is not sufficient and a comprehensive assessment is too expensive or not needed.

3. c **Rationale**: The last and most important step is to report the results, including the implications and recommendations. If the data are not reported, community awareness and changes cannot be achieved.

4. c **Rationale**: Community health nurses work with families and groups to encourage people to take responsibility for their own health care.

5. c **Rationale**: Cultural differences are population variables. Health needs vary among subcultural and ethnic populations.

True/False questions

1. b **Rationale**: The "Windshield Survey" is a familiarization assessment, it is not comprehensive.

2. a **Rationale**: The "location myth" defines a nurse's practice soley by where the nurse practices, not by the scope of the role.

3. b **Rationale**: There are six levels of clients: individuals, families, groups, subpopulations, populations, and communities.

4. a **Rationale**: Any community has all three of these dimensions.

5. a **Rationale**: The problem-oriented assessment focuses on one problem and all assessment data is collected in relation to that problem.

Chapter 10

Multiple-choice questions

1. a **Rationale**: In a childbirth preparation class the primary focus is on learning how to go through childbirth as prepared as possible. A secondary focus would be the support of others.

2. d **Rationale**: The senior citizens planning a health fair are meeting for a specific purpose or task which is their main focus.

3. b **Rationale**: An Alateen group is an example of a support group. They are meeting to give each other support to enable them to cope with alcoholic family members.

4. a **Rationale**: Several factors can block cohesiveness of a group. Open membership makes it difficult for a group to stabilize norms. When members move into and out of a group rapidly, it is almost impossible to establish cohesiveness.

5. a **Rationale**: Maintenance roles are behaviors that promote effective working relationships and a climate of cohesiveness. The gatekeeper helps to keep the channels of communication open and facilitates participation of other members.

True/False questions

1. a **Rationale**: The goal of a learning group is to change behaviors of the members.

2. b **Rationale**: These are the purposes of a support group. In a socialization group the purpose is to help learn new social roles.

3. b **Rationale**: Psychotherapy groups are formed to promote the health of people with emotional disturbances. Task-oriented groups form to accomplish a specific task.

4. a **Rationale**: Small groups go through developmental phases of dependence, counterdependence and interdependence.

5. b **Rationale**: Group termination is important and termination criteria need to be spelled out by the leader at the beginning of the group formation and reinforced during the group functioning.

Chapter 11

Multiple-choice questions

1. a **Rationale**: Interaction is a necessary component of the nursing process in order for it to be effective. It is the relationship between the nurse and client that involves reciprocal influence and exchange.

2. c **Rationale**: Community health nurses look for evidence of all kinds of needs that relate to or influence clients' levels of wellness. Needs cover the whole length of the health-illness continuum and the total person.

3. a **Rationale**: Gathering all the data that will assist the nurse in making a nursing diagnosis makes up the assessment process of the nursing process.

4. b **Rationale**: The desired outcomes described as goals are the measurable terms into which the needs of clients must be translated, to give direction to the nursing care plan.

5. b **Rationale**: The primary data source is the client. Anything the client says, does or produces. All other sources of data outside of the client is a secondary data source.

True/False questions

1. a **Rationale**: The nursing process is systematic with well thought out sequential steps.

2. b **Rationale**: Many sources of data should make up the data collection phase of the nursing process. Methods such as observation, interviewing, and listening are important sources.

3. b **Rationale**: The nursing diagnosis is dynamic and is always changing throughout the caregiving process since the nursing diagnosis reflects changes in the client's health status.

4. a **Rationale**: The steps in the nursing process repeat over and over as the client is brought to a higher level of wellness.

5. a **Rationale**: Specific standards with which to measure achievement of goals are used in the evaluation process.

Chapter 12

Multiple-choice questions

1. c **Rationale**: The host, agent, and environment make up the three parts of this model. Each of the three have to be present to a certain degree in order for any disease, illness, or injury to exist or happen.

2. d **Rationale**: Epidemiological investigation seeks causative determinants of disease, illness, and injury.

3. b **Rationale**: Comparing persons with and without a certain condition is know as a case-control study. There are other types of epidemiologic studies that are conducted in different ways.

4. b **Rationale**: A community trial is conducted as an experimental study design with large populations. Some of the community receives a treatment while the other part does not. The Kingston/Newberg study is a classic community trial.

5. a **Rationale**: The concept of causality looks for the connections between cause and effect. There is a chain of causality and at times causes may be multiple and complex.

True-false questions

1. a **Rationale**: Epidemiology studies the distribution and causitive determinants of all conditions that occur in populations.

2. b **Rationale**: This definition refers to the term prevalence. Incidence refers to new cases of the problem in a certain period of time.

3. a **Rationale**: Epidemiologic studies follow the research process, and the results of well designed studies contribute to the body of knowledge on a given subject.

4. a **Rationale**: There are several types of immunity. Natural passive immunity occurs through maternal antibody transfer.

5. b **Rationale**: Naturally acquired active immunity comes through host infection; acquiring the immunity naturally by getting the disease.

Chapter 13

Multiple-choice questions

1. a **Rationale**: The seven step process has a message, a sender, a receiver, encoding, a channel, decoding, and a feedback loop. The feedback loop is an important step.

2. b **Rationale**: Selective perception destroys the intent of the original message, whether it is the client or the nurse who has selective perception.

3. d **Rationale**: Shared goals and mutual participation are distinguishing factors of collaboration. Depending on the purpose of collaboration, clients may not be on the team. Each person has defined boundaries and responsibilities. Time to accomplish tasks may or may not change.

4. a **Rationale**: The purpose of brainstorming is to allow all ideas and suggestions to flow naturally. After all ideas are exhausted, discussion begins.

5. d **Rationale**: By facilitating client participation in the decision-making process the client is more apt to follow through with ideas and plans, since they contributed to the formulation of the plan or contract.

True-false questions

1. b **Rationale**: Nearly two-thirds of all messages are transmitted nonverbally.

2. b **Rationale**: Sending and receiving in communication are equally important. Both need to be accurate and clearly transmitted.

3. a **Rationale**: Any manipulation of information distorts the intent of the message and becomes a barrier to effective communication.

4. a **Rationale**: The Delphi Technique is a group decision making process that allows a free flow of ideas from all members before decisions are made.

5. b **Rationale**: A grant proposal is a formal contract. It is written and agreed upon by all parties.

Chapter 14

Multiple-choice questions

1. a **Rationale**: The knowledge level of cognitive learning is the lowest level and the learner can perform repetitive behaviors, such as: to recall, list or name items.

2. c **Rationale**: At the application level of cognitive learning the learner applies information, such as eating well balanced meals.

3. d **Rationale**: Behavioral theory is grounded in stimulus-response behaviors and changes occur in response to a stimuli.

4. c **Rationale**: The teaching process has the steps of interaction, *assessment and diagnosis*, setting goals and objectives, *planning*, teaching (*implementation*), and *evaluation*. The italicized words are the steps of the nursing process.

5. b **Rationale**: The cognitive learning progression is knowledge, comprehension, application, analysis, synthesis, and evaluation.

True/False questions

1. b **Rationale**: The goal of teaching is learning.

2. a **Rationale**: In humanistic theory there is a natural tendency for people to learn. They do so in an encouraging environment.

3. b **Rationale**: Knowledge involves recall, but is the lowest level of cognitive learning.

4. a **Rationale**: Psychomotor learning involves visible, demonstrable, performance skills that require neuromuscular coordination. Infant bathing requires a great deal of coordination to complete. It is a complex psychomotor skill.

5. a **Rationale**: Clients' readiness to learn is affected by their needs, interests, and concerns. Educational background and maturation also influence readiness to learn.

Chapter 15

Multiple-choice questions

1. c **Rationale**: Crisis is described as a temporary event that comes with or without warning and disturbs the equilibrium of a person, group, or community.

2. b **Rationale**: A developmental crisis is defined as a transitional event in a person's normal growth and development, that is disruptive and stressful.

3. a **Rationale**: Refer to Table 15-1, p. 327, see goals and interventions.

4. a **Rationale**: Refer to Table 15-1, p. 327, see phase and goals.

5. d **Rationale**: The stated goal of crisis intervention is to reestablish equilibrium. At the pre-crisis phase preventing the crisis altogether would be the goal.

True/False questions

1. a **Rationale**: A developmental crisis is defined as a transitional event in a person's normal growth and development, that is disruptive and stressful.

2. b **Rationale**: Community health nurses DO intervene at the pre-crisis phase. Refer to Table 15-1, pre-crisis phase.

3. b **Rationale**: All events that disrupt equilibrium in an individual, family, group, or community can be considered a crisis.

4. a **Rationale**: It is during the early portion of the crisis phase, at time of shock or impact, when the client first encounters the crisis situation.

5. b **Rationale**: In the later part of the crisis phase clients begin to use coping strategies of defensive retreat, denial, anger, and bargaining. Shock occurs early in the crisis phase.

Chapter 16

Multiple-choice questions

1. a **Rationale**: "With today's wide variety of family types and structures, the most advanced definition of family may be 'the family is who the client says it is' (Bell and Wright , 1993, p. 391)."

2. b **Rationale**: Families are not closed systems. Their boundaries are semi-permeable, providing protection and preservation of family unity and autonomy while also allowing selective linkage with external associations.

3. a **Rationale**: Family values become powerful determinants of family beliefs, feelings, thoughts, and actions.

4. c **Rationale**: A nuclear dyad consists of a husband and wife living as a couple who either have no children or whose children are launched. A nuclear family is made up of a husband, wife, and children living together.

5. d **Rationale**: Homeless families are increasing in society today. Drugs, alcohol, increased cost of living and housing, and divorce all contribute to this new nontraditional family.

True/False questions

1. a **Rationale**: Families are increasingly nontraditional with many new types and structures which causing a broadening of the definition of family.

2. b **Rationale**: A family does not have to be a group or have children. Newer definitions include one member families.

3. b **Rationale**: The blended family is a relatively new family structure occurring more frequently due to the high divorce and remarriage rate in the United States. The blended family is so common today that it now can be considered traditional.

4. a **Rationale**: There are six functions typical of families in the United states today. They are affection, security, identity, affiliation, socialization, and controls.

5. b **Rationale**: Clearly defined limits are appropriate for the young child. By the time they are teenagers, controls have shifted to self control and focus on the relationships between family members and outsiders.

Chapter 17

Multiple-choice questions

1. b **Rationale**: An ecomap diagrams a family's relationships to its external environment. Lines are drawn to indicate connections to other systems, arrows signify the direction of energy or flow of resources, and absence of lines indicates a lack of connections.

2. a **Rationale**: The Level II family is at a higher level of functioning than the Level I family. They remain disorganized and have limited ability to trust. However, the family functions at a higher level than the chaotic Level I family and functions lower than the Level III family (a fairly normal family with more than its share of problems).

3. d **Rationale**: In the example cited, the nurse works with the family as a whole, not with individuals, to change behaviors. The family participates in the activities to achieve family goals. The other answer choices are inherent in the nurse's work with all families.

4. d **Rationale**: The interactional framework portrays the family unit as a union of interacting personalities. It describes the family in terms of its internal relationships; emphasizing communication, roles, conflict, coping patterns, and decision-making processes. It does not consider the family's interaction with its external environment.

5. a **Rationale**: Making an accurate family assessment takes time. The nurse should not use obtrusive questionnaire techniques, or take notes in the family's presence. It is better to keep notes from several visits with the family, and observe the family as a group during some family activity. The nurse should collect both quantitative and qualitative data.

True-false questions

1. a **Rationale**: Genograms depict generations of family members and their relationships to one another. No other outside systems are displayed. Most genograms include at least three generations but may go as far back in history as is known.

2. b **Rationale**: The Level V family is the mature family and rarely needs the services of a community health nurse. They function independent of the services of a community health nurse. They have rich resources and maintain a high level of wellness as a family.

3. b **Rationale**: A healthy family needs to establish links with the community and cannot remain isolated. Some families exist in isolation but they do not display all the characteristics of a healthy family.

4. a **Rationale**: The developmental framework follows growth and developmental patterns similar to the life cycle perspective, which follows a predictable pattern of development.

5. a **Rationale**: This is fundamental to the work with any client in any setting. The nurse can only begin to build from the point where the family is developmentally, educationally, or emotionally.

Chapter 18

Multiple-choice questions

1. d **Rationale**: Infant mortality dropped to 9.2 per 1000 live births in 1990 (statistical Abstracts of the U.S., 1993). However infant mortality continues to rank higher in infant mortality than 21 other countries, including Japan, France, Italy, and the Scandinavian countries.

2. c **Rationale**: Teaching is the major focus of community health nursing intervention during the antepartum and postpartum periods. The nurse introduces new information or reinforces clients' existing knowledge of pregnancy, labor and delivery, postpartum health considerations, and infant care.

3. b **Rationale**: Numerous projects have either failed or been ineffective because the targeted populations were assessed incompletely, or not involved in the planning process.

4. a **Rationale**: The health of infants can be dramatically affected by maternal consumption of alcohol. The pregnancy itself can be threatened. However, the most devastating consequence of alcohol consumption during pregnancy, for the surviving fetus, is being born with FAE or FAS, both of which compromise the intellectual functioning of the infant/child.

5. b **Rationale**: The most common side effect on the fetus from a mother who smokes during the pregnancy is a lowered birth weight. Newborns weigh an average of 200 gms lower at birth in some studies. Other studies have shown that there is a greater incidence of stillbirths, spontaneous abortions, and perinatal mortality in pregnancies where women smoke.

True/False questions

1. a **Rationale**: this is the goal of self-help groups. If clients are able to regain a sense of identity and control, they are able to promote their own health and prevent crises in their lives. It is a form of primary prevention which eliminates the need for secondary or tertiary prevention.

2. a **Rationale**: Infants born to mothers who use alcohol during pregnancy are three times more likely to suffer the effects of FAE than FAS. Both are irreversible and have effects that compromise intellect, growth and development, facial and cranial formation, behavior, and feeding patterns.

3. b **Rationale**: The HIV virus does exit in breast milk and can transmit the virus to the infant (Ellerbrock and Rogers, 1990).

4. b **Rationale**: Fetal exposure to drugs taken by women during pregnancy is a major health problem in the United States. There are over 375,000 drug exposed infants and 10,000-15,000 infants born to drug dependent women each year in the United States.

5. a **Rationale**: Funds come to the states from the federal government. The states distribute it to the receivers of care through services delivered at the local level. These providers include health departments, clinics, community centers, and health care practitioners offices.

Chapter 19

Multiple-choice questions

1. d **Rationale**: Vital statistics show that for children ages 1-14 accidents are the leading cause of death. For children of all ages accidents are a major cause of death.

2. d **Rationale**: Schoolchildren's diets are usually high in sugar and fat. Caloric intake often involves overeating of "empty" calories.

3. c **Rationale**: Answer (a) is a prevention activity, while answers (b) and (d) are health promotion interventions. Case finding, and reporting of communicable diseases protect children from illness.

4. a **Rationale**: Motor vehicle accidents are the leading cause of death in white males and females. Other types of accidents are second. Homicide is the leading cause of death for non-white males and females (with firearm violence the leading cause of death for the 15-19 year old black male), and motor vehicle accidents are second.

5. d **Rationale**: The child with ADD displays signs and symptoms of a quieter nature than the children with ADHD. Activities such as not listening, losing things, not paying attention, and day dreaming are common. See Table 19-1.

True/False questions

1. a **Rationale**: The school-age child is exposed to more people, having new life events which increases exposure to others. Due to physical and emotional changes, acute infections are most prevalent in this group.

2. b **Rationale**: Learning disabilities and behavior problems affect between 10 - 15% of school-age children.

3. a **Rationale**: This is true for the population mentioned. Firearm violence is ten times more prevalent in black males ages 15-19 than for white males.

4. a **Rationale**: According to the U.S. Statistical Abstracts, 1993; the incidence has doubled in the 20 years from 1970-1990.

5. b **Rationale**: This is not true. The actual percentage is 60% with a female ratio 2 to 1.

Chapter 20

Multiple-choice questions

1. c **Rationale**: Ergonomic factors include the potential physiological and psychological stressors on the worker created by space allotments, tools, and physical positions workers must assume.

2. d **Rationale**: Farmers are potentially exposed to all of these factors. In the other occupations mentioned only 1 or 2 of the factors may be an issue in their work settings. However all the workers mentioned may be exposed to other categories of environmental health factors.

3. b **Rationale**: OSHA assures safe and healthful working conditions for men and women through development and enforcement of regulations and standards, maintenance of safety and health statistics, and worker safety education. The other answer choices are parts of other significant health and safety acts passed in the United States.

4. a **Rationale**: A condition such a silicosis takes 15 years to develop. Some cases of mesothelioma (asbestos lung) may not become apparent for 25 years. Uranium exposure produces lung cancer in about 1/6 of workers in approximately 20 years, and more than 12 percent of coal mine workers show evidence of pneumoconiosis (black lung).

5. c **Rationale**: The Americans with Disabilities Act has many facets. One aspect is to prevent discrimination against qualified workers. The workplace also has to make necessary physical changes to accommodate the disabled. The other answer choices are parts of other significant health and safety acts passed in the United States.

True/False questions

1. b **Rationale**: There are fewer injuries and deaths at work now than ten years ago. The numbers have decreased from 20 million workers injured to 17 million, and 99,000 deaths instead of 100,000.

2. b **Rationale**: This is a responsibility of OSHA, not NIOSH. NIOSH is the administrative, training, and research branch of occupational health and safety. OSHA is the regulatory and enforcing branch.

3. a **Rationale**: This is a responsibility of OSHA and part of its regulatory and enforcing mandates.

4. b **Rationale**: This act ensures that only necessary information be collected on individuals by federal agencies. It has nothing to do with numbers and types of bathroom facilities in the workplace.

5. a **Rationale**: The Social Security Act of 1935 was the first act to consider the financial needs of our aged, blind and disabled citizens. Since that date these populations have been eligible for financial aid to increase their ability to be self sufficient.

Chapter 21

Multiple-choice questions

1. b **Rationale**: Services for the elderly should be proactive. Nurses should design interventions that maximize nursing resources and provide the greatest benefit to elderly clients.

2. a **Rationale**: Lowered blood pressure, know as postural hypotension, when arising quickly, can produce vertigo and cause a fall. Forty percent of older adults have blood pressure high enough to be considered hypertensive. Black females have the highest rates of hypertension.

3. c **Rationale**: The practice of gerontics safeguards, extends, and enhances health care and the comfort of elders. Geriatrics focuses on abnormal conditions, and gerontology is broad and multidisciplined. Case management is a coordinated system of care throughout an illness.

4. a **Rationale**: The concept of continuing care centers is to provide housing, services, and health care as needed for an aging adult. A 70 year old resident may live independently with minimal services, while a 95 year old resident may live in a room with a roommate and receive all services and medical care offered.

5. d **Rationale**: Reducing suicides among older adults, especially white males, is one of the goals of "Healthy People 2000." The other answer choices are worthwhile, but are not identified as specific areas to focus on in the Healthy People 2000 document.

True/False questions

1. b **Rationale**: Senility is not a legitimate medical diagnosis, even though it has been a widely used term even by professionals. Confusion or dementia may stem from problems such as drug interaction, depression, metabolic disorders, nutritional deficiencies, or certain cerebral disorders such as hematomas, tumors, and sensory deprivation. However, this confusion or dementia affects only a small portion of elders.

2. b **Rationale**: Healthy elders continue to be active and involved. Activity produces the best psychological climate for older adults.

3. b **Rationale**: All people benefit from continuous exercise that is designed with age and ability in mind. A sedentary life-style is not healthy for any person.

4. a **Rationale**: The loneliness many older adults experiences after the loss of a loved one can be so deep that if affects their will to live. Surviving older adults may neglect their own health or intentionally engage in activities to cause their own death. This can be prevented through nursing intervention (see Chapter 15 on crisis prevention).

5. a **Rationale**: By maintaining their independence, older adults promote their self-esteem and preserve their dignity. Providing services in the homes of older adults will help them stay independent as long as possible.

Chapter 22

Multiple-choice questions

1. c **Rationale**: The other services in answer choices (a), (b), or (d) were not founded by Lillian Wald in 1893, however they did exist.

2. a **Rationale**: With the advent of Medicare and Medicaid the payment source for older adult care changed along with the advent of standards for determining client eligibility. Physicians direct the care and the home care model is based on the medical model.

3. a **Rationale**: The one sure thing about our health care delivery system is that change is inevitable and the future is uncertain. Technical care will continue to increase in the home, home care will continue to grow, and the model used now is destined to change as our nation looks more seriously at a national health insurance plan.

4. b **Rationale**: Getting feedback from discharged clients is one way of improving care and is a tool used in a quality management program.

5. d **Rationale**: The two populations differ, however the needs of home care clients have been determined as skilled according to Medicare or Medicaid guidelines and the population is older. The needs of community health nursing clients are as varied and as important as those of the home care client but are not covered under Medicare or Medicaid.

True/False questions

1. a **Rationale**: Cost containment is the motivation behind the dramatic home care movement.

2. b **Rationale**: The largest segment of home care clients are men and women over the age of 65. Two-thirds of the older clients are women. The number of mothers and infants receiving home care has increased due to the shorter postpartum stay most hospitals offer, and insurance companies pay for, but their numbers are small in comparison.

3. a **Rationale**: It began with Lillian Wald in New York City in 1893. It grew slowly until the early 1980s when the movements growth accelerated.

4. a **Rationale**: This is a growing group of home care clients. AIDS clients can be cared for at home for extended periods of time due to their ability to provide their own self-care. Treatments administered in the home can prolong and promote the quality of their lives.

5. b **Rationale**: Medicare is selective in the services it covers; it determines the actions that are skilled and cover many of them. However, many older adults have transportation and custodial care needs, which are not covered by Medicare.

Chapter 23

Multiple-choice questions

1. a **Rationale**: Gonorrhea is the most frequently reported communicable disease. Syphilis has decreased in incidence in recent years. AIDS, although widespread and with lethal consequences, is far lower in occurrence than gonorrhea. Although tuberculosis has had recent upsurges in incidence since the 1980s, there are still fewer cases of it than gonorrhea. For actual numbers of cases refer to USPHS, 1991.

2. b **Rationale**: There are many factors that interplay in the AIDS epidemic, however sexual behavior, illegal drug use and end-of -life issues are three major ones. The multidimensional services, caregiver attitudes, and perhaps legal violations of drug abuse that surround AIDS clients, complicate caregiving. The caregiver is not at risk if universal preccautions are used. There is no cure for AIDS and the AIDS client generally does not have negative attitudes towards caregivers.

3. d **Rationale**: The three goals are: 1) promoting general health and resilience, 2) preventing infections of all sorts, and 3) delaying the onset of clinical symptoms with antiviral therapy.

4. b **Rationale**: Classification III is the classification for TB disease. Clients have had exposure, a positive skin test, and positive chest x-ray and/or sputum tests.

5. d **Rationale**: Administering flu vaccine is the only primary prevention example. The other three are secondary in that they are all looking for disease, hopefully in the early stages, so treatment can commence promptly.

True/False questions

1. a **Rationale**: If the entire population of the world were to be tested for tuberculosis, one billon people would have a positive PPD, indicating a TB infection.

2. b **Rationale**: Due to a decreased immune system, AIDS clients will give a false negative on their TB skin test. Twenty-five percent of AIDS clients also have TB.

3. b **Rationale**: Passive immunity is short term resistance to disease-causing organisms. Acquired can be life-long.

4. a **Rationale**: If treatment is not completed, the organisms become stronger and may mutate and begin to resist traditional therapy regimens.

5. b **Rationale**: TB kills three million people each year, more than any other single infectious disease (USPHS, 1991). Anti-TB medications have been around since the 1940's.

Chapter 24

Multiple-choice questions

1. b **Rationale**: The damage to the family's home by a tornado was a one time problem and constitutes a temporary homeless situation. The other answer choices depict clients who have behaviors that would make them episodically or chronically homeless.

2. c **Rationale**: The fact that a client has been laid off from work, or abuses drugs and alcohol intermittently, might put him/her into the situation of being episodically homeless. The client with no skills or resources who abuses alcohol is in a situation of being chronically homeless.

3. d **Rationale**: The National Institute of Mental Health has targeted three goals: 1) to determine reliable estimates of the incidence and prevalence of mental disorders, 2) to explore possible causes, and 3) to assist with planning and development of mental health services.

4. b **Rationale**: This is an example of a behavioral factor. Others include, job burnout, being an unwanted child, or low self-esteem. The other answer

choices fall into the other three causal categories: sociocultural, biological, and environmental.

5. a **Rationale**: Self-destructive tendencies are a characteristic of a drug dependent person. Other characteristics include underachievement, lonliness, social conflicts, fear of closeness, and identity problems. Levels of intelligence do not affect drug dependency, nor do people need to take more than one drug to be drug dependent.

True/False questions

1. b **Rationale**: Thirty to forty percent of the homeless are mentally ill (Berne, 1990).

2. a **Rationale**: These are the four categories and there are variables within each domain of vulnerability.

3. a **Rationale**: Suggestions of nursing actions to eliminate environmental variables include assessing for environmental risk factors and informing consumers and agencies about the impact of the environment, in addition to advocating for a healthier environment.

4. b **Rationale**: 7-15% of drug abusers are chemically addicted (Peele, 1985).

5. a **Rationale**: Although there are still more single men who are homeless, an alarming change in the statistics of the homeless is that the fastest growing group is mothers with young children.

Chapter 25

Multiple-Choice Questions

1. d **Rationale**: In Lewin's change model there are three steps of unfreezing the old behavior, implementing the change, and then refreezing the new change in place to integrated it into the system.

2. c **Rationale**: Normative-reeducative strategies not only give information but also directly influence people to change attitudes and behaviors.

3. a **Rationale**: The autocratic leadership style uses the power of the position to influence followers. The autocratic leader gives orders and expects followers to obey.

4. b **Rationale**: The participative leader values the input from group members and involves them in the decision-making process.

5. a **Rationale**: This base of power influences by rewarding or providing something of value in exchange for compliance.

True/False Questions

1. b **Rationale**: Evolutionary change tends to be gradual and requires adjustment on an incremental basis.

2. b **Rationale**: At times, leaders need to be risk takers and proceed with the necessary changes that improve outcomes.

3. a **Rationale**: The community health nurse is an influence on the community's health and should be a positive one.

4. a **Rationale**: Unfreezing is the first step of Lewin's three step change model.

5. a **Rationale**: There are four criteria for effective planned change and this is one of them. Planned change has purpose and occurs intentionally.

Chapter 26

Multiple-Choice Questions

1. a **Rationale**: The conceptual model clarifies the focus and direction of the study and looks at the world in terms of nursing's major concerns.

2. b **Rationale**: Inferential studies are used to imply that relationships seen in the group of individuals studied (sample) are likely to exist in the larger group of concern (population).

3. a **Rationale**: A true experiment is characterized by manipulation of one of the variables, randomization, and the use of a control group.

4. b **Rationale**: An overview of recent literature assists the researcher in getting direction and focus on a topic of interest. This is followed by an in-depth study of literature (no more than five years old).

5. c **Rationale**: Opinion polls, or asking subjects for their opinions on topics, is considered valid information to gather. Gossip, hearsay, and rumors have no place in legitimate research.

True/False Questions

1. b **Rationale**: Research studies can be done by a multidisciplinary team of colleagues or by one investigator. Involvement of others is based on size and comprehensiveness of the study.

2. b **Rationale**: All eight steps of the research must be followed. None of the steps are more important than others.

3. b **Rationale**: Both quantitative and qualitative research has value. Their focus on subjects is different and the findings complement each other.

4. a **Rationale**: True experimental studies are expensive (financial, time, and subject availability). Due to lack of all necessary resources many experimental studies are developed as quasi- experimental studies.

5. a **Rationale**: The tools needed to consistently measure what is intended to be measured in the given population. There are tests that can be conducted on the tools to determine validity and reliability before using them.

Chapter 27

Multiple-Choice Questions

1. c **Rationale**: Through the use of quality indicators as a quality assurance tool, facilitation of ongoing self-evaluation occurs.

2. a **Rationale**: Accessibility of an agency is demonstrated if it is readily involved with its population on a timely basis despite financial, cultural, emotional, and geographic barriers that may be present.

3. b **Rationale**: Agency efficiency is determined by how it makes use of its resources, finds new resources, and then delivers care in an efficient manner.

4. d **Rationale**: Standards measure health care activities on three levels: structure, process, and outcome. Criteria are measurable indicators that standards or goals have been achieved.

5. c **Rationale**: A quality circle is a participative management style developed in Japan forty years ago and is used in successful businesses. It is a concept that has come to the health care delivery arena and shares the responsibility for decisions among management and staff.

True/False Questions

1. b **Rationale**: The Donabedian model looks at structure, process, and outcome as its framework.

2. a **Rationale**: The four models described in Chapter 27 are based on the Donabedian model that looks at structure, process, and outcome as its framework.

3. a **Rationale**: "Quality is not an event, it's a way of life to conduct business, an ongoing quest for excellence." (Kirk and Hoesing, 1990, p. 3.)

4. a **Rationale**: Quality indicators are used as markers to determine if goals have been met. They are quality-focused. Quality indicator is defined in the text within Chapter 27 and in the glossary.

5. b **Rationale**: Retrospective review is conducted on closed charts in an organization. Concurrent review is conducted on charts of clients presently being served.

Chapter 28

Multiple-Choice Questions

1. a **Rationale**: Health policy should reflect a community's values and should not only be created for certain groups such as the influential or the poor. It needs to come from the people within the community.

2. c **Rationale**: Regulatory health policy regulates or licenses services or people providing services in the community. Distributive health policy subsidizes nursing education, benefits the needy, and allocates resources among and between groups.

3. b **Rationale**: In the United States a greater percentage of income is spent on health care than is spent in any other country and the amount keeps increasing. Other issues, such as accessibility, quality, and special groups of uninsured and underinsured, are significant, but cost remains the most troubling issue.

4. c **Rationale**: The legislative process is long and detailed and is initiated at the local level; taking skill, power, money, and patience to pursue it. The processes are similar at the state and federal levels.

5. c **Rationale**: The political activist role should not be added to a nurse's role description nor do nurses have the time to become watchdogs to legislators. No one should be in control of health policy at any level. The nurse as a change agent, however, needs to be involved and influential in the community's political arena.

True/False Questions

1. a **Rationale**: Political decisions are made by those people most interested in the issues. These people are referred to as stakeholders, meaning people who have a personal interest in the decision.

2. b **Rationale**: Health policies are made at the federal or state levels and affect the local level.

3. b **Rationale**: Health policies are highly influenced by special interest groups.

4. a **Rationale**: The stages of policy adoption include these four steps.

5. a **Rationale**: This is most frequently where change begins. A small group of people with a special interest lobby for changes, gain support, and influence legislators to back a policy change.